WHAT DO YOU
EXPECT...?

Some people are happier and healthier than before...

...some more than they were expecting

Some people want their stories to be told so others
might benefit too.

Mary Ratcliffe

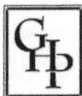

Grosvenor House
Publishing Limited

The right of Mary Ratcliffe to be identified as the author of this
work has been asserted by her in accordance with Section 78
of the Copyright, Designs and Patents Act 1988

The book cover picture is copyright to ©olly/Fotolia

This book is published by
Grosvenor House Publishing Ltd
28-30 High Street, Guildford, Surrey, GU1 3EL.
www.grosvenorhousepublishing.co.uk

Lesserian Curative Hypnotherapy™ and
LCH® are registered trademarks and
use of them is subject to UK law.

A CIP record for this book
is available from the British Library

ISBN 978-1-78148-713-6

For Michael

Reviews

An amazing read, really had me transfixed to want to know the outcome of each case study.

I can't thank you enough for your help in changing my life. If I hadn't picked up your card that day I would very possibly not be here now, my life was really spiralling out of control and I had no way of knowing how to get it back. I'm so glad to be living proof that there can be an alternative to years of medicine and therapy.

Cathy

I've read it and I'm happy to approve my section. To be honest I've enjoyed going through the experience again. I'd forgotten what it was like.

Steve

I found it very interesting and enjoyed it more than your first book.

Clare

I've finally finished reading your latest version. I can't think of anything to improve it and I'm very happy for you to send it out to others. Well done.

Bill

As a client of Mary I have personally experienced the life changing magic that LCH can manifest. This second book has shown parallel examples except for the final story of a gluten allergy which completely blew my mind. I think the only thing more surprising is that it is under researched and over looked by modern day science. More research needs to be carried out in this field to help others.

Simon

We are living in extra-ordinary times. Science is meeting ancient and part-forgotten wisdoms and teachings, and a beautifully profound union is taking place before our very eyes. LCH is a perfect example of this phenomenon. Via what could be described as a stunning fusion of logic and intuition, LCH therapists and their clients are experiencing astonishing results.

Mary's second book, 'What do you expect... ?' is another delve into the wondrous world of LCH. In her own unmistakably honest, quaint and gentle style, via the fascinating accounts of her work and the sharing of personal methodologies, Mary treats us to a deeper insight into LCH. This includes how her clients have benefited holistically in addition to the issues for which they initially sought help.

As a potential or current client, this book provides a most useful companion to the explanations and descriptions provided by the therapist. As a practising LCH therapist, or one who is considering following this path, it can be read, enjoyed and utilised in numerous ways to further understanding and develop skills.

On a more personal note, this book is a huge inspiration for me to continue my own journey into the magical world of LCH, to gently push the boundaries of what can be accomplished further still for the benefit of each individual who seeks freedom from issues and problems that prevent them from shining their own, unique light into the world. When people are liberated in this way, they empower others to shine too.

In Mary's own words, LCH really is the 'gift that keeps on giving'.

Katherine M Harris – Lesserian™ Curative Hypnotherapist, Usui and Karuna Reiki Master Teacher

I found this book very readable and informative. Mary writes really clearly, explaining LCH theory in a way that makes it very easy to understand. Her case studies are compelling. And I love her use of imagery and metaphor.

As a (non-LCH) therapist, my first introduction to LCH was through Mary's first book. The approach makes sense to me as a highly sophisticated and effective process for clearing the underlying subconscious decisions that drive present day problems. I will be recommending this book to colleagues and clients wishing to understand more about this process.

Pauline Brumwell - Psychotherapeutic Counsellor and Hypnotherapist.

I've just finished reading your book and I've been totally gripped by it! I love the format - it made it so easy to read and I was fascinated by the case studies. I really had no idea what to expect, but I feel as though I have learned so much and want to know more!

Before reading your book I was apprehensive about having hypnotherapy, even though I had considered it in the past, but I now feel better informed and would be more confident about trying it in the future.

It has certainly made me think!

I am now reading and enjoying your first book too!

Chris Walker - Maths Teacher/Tutor

A good follow up. Made me think of the phrase "If it ain't broke, don't fix it" BUT the problem with us humans and our minds is: we don't always KNOW it's broke; even when we do, we usually don't know WHICH is the part (or parts) that's broke; and even if we know it's broke and which bit's broke, we don't know HOW to fix it.

If, like me, you're one of those people who've always questioned what REALLY brought about improvement or cure: Mary's account of her clients' experiences shows that accepting and enjoying a good result is much more sensible than questioning how it happened. There's some wonderful magic to be found in mystery.

Harry Parker - BSc (Hons) Behavioural Sciences

This book provides a great insight in to real life examples of how LCH can help, from serious habits to medical illnesses and psychological issues. It gives clear explanations with great analogies to how the subconscious is at the helm of some of our problems. It should be read by everyone that has related issues, including sceptics.

It's impossible for me to understand why science has not pushed LCH in to common public health. This book details the limitations of a placebo explanation by recording multiple cures to previously unknown issues from the same treatment. It's a very powerful read and a must for anyone interested in how our mind controls our health. If you are conscious, you should read this book!

Gavin Marriott - Software Engineer

Contents

Foreword

Discovering the 'why behind the why', understanding the reason why the subconscious has developed the reaction (symptom), working efficiently through all the many and varied events, incidents and circumstances in a person's life which have played some part or other in the creation of the problem – this can seem a daunting prospect for both therapist and patient alike. And, at first glance, it does indeed seem like seeking a very tiny needle in an exceedingly large haystack.

This is not, however, the case. There is a definite end-point to work from. If the subconscious has created a symptom or behaviour for a reason then that reason, that information, has to exist and by following the logical path from effect back to cause, the relevant information can be methodically identified and dealt with.

So it may be a large haystack and it may be a small needle but if you already have the one end of that thread, it is a straightforward matter to just follow it simply and efficiently back to the other end and retrieve that needle.

This book sets out to give examples of how that process affected (and continues to affect) those who have undergone LCH therapy. It does not attempt to explain how to apply the treatment – that is not its purpose. This is not a book about LCH therapy nor is it even about LCH therapists – it is how one therapist has used the understanding and skills she's been taught to deepen her knowledge and insight and use her own abilities, perceptions, attitude and experiences to apply all this for the benefit of those who receive treatment from her.

In this book, Mary Ratcliffe explains how the co-operation between therapist and patient is required, how effortlessly this can be achieved and why the collaboration between therapist and subconscious significantly reduces any chance of the kind of adverse reaction many other therapies or interventions have to navigate.

Through these pages, the author shows how a trained therapist can use this logical, methodical system to help people to achieve more than even they thought possible. The joy that is gained from helping people to live their lives more comfortably and contentedly shines through clearly – and allows the reader a glimpse of that wonderful sense of purpose and satisfaction we therapists can so easily take for granted.

Whether they are described as conditions, symptoms, issues, syndromes, difficulties, complaints, disorders, ailments or other maladies; the case studies are not about problem people, they are about people with problems.

No one should ever feel ashamed to need or to have treatment – even if it were possible for a mere mortal to achieve perfection, as we go through life our perceptions change, our views expand and our wants, needs and desires alter. As our lives change, as we wish to gain more, learn more, achieve more, *be* more – we may find things more difficult than anticipated or simply that our expectations of ourselves are self-limiting and that, actually, we could do even more. Don't we owe it to ourselves and to those who our lives touch to do something about that?

We each have this amazing gift of life right now. None of us know how long we can benefit from it or what may be in store for us – but isn't a gift supposed to be enjoyed? One can keep a gift safely tucked away, carefully contained and rarely used but isn't its very preciousness in the fact that it can be stretched, applied, enjoyed, employed, utilised in whatever way we choose? To my mind, it is empowering, it is deserved – it is right that we make the most of the gift of life. The more content/happier we are within ourselves, the more we benefit those around us – physically, emotionally, mentally.

The case studies revealed in this publication show how changing the limiting Core Beliefs not only allows a person to be free of the condition for which they sought treatment, but also the impact on other, often unexpected, areas of their lives. We can all be rather short-sighted when it comes to ourselves, we put up with aches and pains, we dismiss allergies, fears or negativity as being 'just me', something we have to just accept and work around. So many times, in my own practice, we near the end of treatment for one problem and the patient will remark on some other symptom or difficulty which seems to have magically disappeared – and they begin to think of other ways their lives could be further improved. A whole new world of possibilities and opportunity opens up for them.

My thanks go to Mary Ratcliffe for writing this book. If just one person decides to enrich their lives by having a course of treatment or becoming an LCH therapist because of it, then this book will have done its job and the ripples of one life changed will spread out across unknown distances for the benefit of so many more.

Helen Lesser. Birmingham April 2014.

Acknowledgements

It takes a whole village to raise a child and it took a whole crowd of generous, patient, encouraging and enthusiastic people to help a hypnotherapist go back to the computer, time and again, until this creature with a mind of its own was nurtured through those difficult in-between years from the first spark of an idea to a grown-up ready to face the world.

Helen Lesser created the current form of the therapy itself out of Phase 1 which her late father, David Lesser invented, and together, they gave me a huge fertile landscape to explore and describe. Over the years covered by this book, Helen has kept me on my toes with messages about my writing that tell me she knows I can do better, and I've been so happy to discover that she is so often right.

Katherine Harris, a colleague and fellow hypnotherapist, spent many hours with a fine tooth comb for the detail and a clear and insightful mind for the broader picture, the clarity of explanations, the removal of unintended ambiguities. She is also responsible for some of the quotations which she has generously allowed me to include. I think she uses some of mine from time to time, but I've not been keeping score, so if I'm in her debt on that trade-off, then that's yet another reason to send her a huge thank you. She has contributed so much by being there all those times when I needed to revive my self-belief.

Emma Parker has nothing to do with hypnotherapy and yet took on my request to read a draft and give me feedback with a conscientious and meticulous response that totally took me by surprise. Among her suggestions are some that, I believe, have helped make a significant difference to the readability of the final version. She has shown her belief in me and what I'm doing and I've grown a few emotional inches as a result.

The following people are just a few from the crowd who have done some or all of the following - read drafts, sent me encouragement, given me their support and much more. A simple thank-you is just not enough but I hope they all know, whether named here or not, how much I appreciate each and every ounce of energy and interest they've so generously given me. They include: -

Michael Cardis - Gwen Blundell - Chris Walker - Pauline Brumwell – Harry Parker – Vanita Grad – Steve Phillips – William Broom – Barbara and Bill Hull – Tracie Jarvis – Angie Broad – Anne McLean

And none of this would have happened without four people I can only name as Clare, Cathy, Steve and Bill. You, alone, know who you are. Thank you so much for making this possible.

CHAPTER 1

Imagine there's another person on the chair next to you, and that's your subconscious mind

Let me start with a couple of introductions, or reminders if you already met them from the pages of my first book, my musings about the subconscious mind 'What if it really is... ?'

Pat and Chris are old friends of mine and I'd lost touch with them both over the years, but we had got back together a couple of years after I qualified in Lesserian™ Curative Hypnotherapy (LCH). 'What if it really is... ?' includes my interpretation of LCH, the theory behind it and how it works with the subconscious for the benefit of the client. It also includes some personal information about treatment I've received and some of the differences that treatment has made to me and to my life.

What is LCH?

In case you're totally new to LCH, this is just a very brief summary to help us get started. Much more detail will follow. LCH is a form of hypnotherapy where the therapist works with the subconscious mind to resolve the underlying cause of the symptom, condition or issue that the client consciously wishes to dispose of.

Just like the way the dentist focuses on fixing the tooth decay or gum disease or abscess that is causing the pain, the LCH therapist focuses on the subconscious cause of the habit or phobia or anxiety or whatever is bothering the client. Once resolved at the roots, the toothache or the client's symptom tends to go away all on its own without any further need for pain-killers or other symptom-management.

Who are Pat and Chris?

Pat is considering training to be some kind of therapist and, so far, is finding LCH intriguing, has read the College's prospectus, but is a bit nervous and would like a bit more help in the decision. A career change is a big one for anyone, so more information, as long as it's honest and unbiased, can improve the likelihood that the best choice will be made in the long run. It's not a deliberation to be rushed.

Chris is considering having some treatment for a fear of driving, a peanut allergy and Obsessive Compulsive Disorder (O.C.D.) and again, a bit more accurate and wide-reaching information could lead to a more informed choice and a more beneficial outcome.

Pat and Chris are helping me get my thoughts and ideas together. We have just re-read 'What if it really is... ?' and we are all wondering what has changed since then for all of us, and for the people I have treated. We also wonder what questions were raised and left hanging around, rather than answered or clarified there.

The two books are complete in themselves, each looking at the subject from a specific but different angle. If you haven't read 'What if it really is... ?' then you might find questions forming in your own mind from this book because some of the foundation ideas are not explored in detail here. If your curiosity is aroused, your enquiring mind intrigued to look more into the theory, then 'What if...' is my first suggestion of where to look for some more food for thought.

Both books are written in an informal rather than an academic style, with no references, no index, no appendices and no footnotes. There is no single writing style that suits everyone's taste or reading preference. You might want to read it as if it were a novel and simply allow the various messages to come through as they occur in the story.

If you'd prefer a bit more structure, to give you an idea of what's to follow, we start with some general information about the subconscious mind and hypnotherapy. We then explore the experiences of 4 people who have received LCH therapy. At the mid-point, I digress into some details about my training and early years as a therapist. Following on from the 4 case studies, I look more deeply into the longer term effect the treatment I've received has had on me personally. We finish with a few questions we might want to consider for the future.

In 'What if it really is… ?', I refer to the people on the receiving end of treatment mainly as patients rather than clients. There are various pros and cons of each reference and I don't believe either is universally better than the other, so in the interest of balance, this time, Pat and Chris and I refer to those people mainly as clients.

What does a client need to know?

Pat: *How do you explain the subconscious to a new client? If they arrive with no knowledge of your work and your theories, if they haven't read anything you've written and you only have about 30 minutes to get the whole idea across to them, what do you say? Let's imagine someone coming to you for treatment, they just found you on the internet because they searched for hypnotherapy or hypnotherapist. Let's imagine they don't want to, can't be bothered to, or don't have time to read a book about it.*

Me: That's quite realistic. It's pretty much how it is for most of the people who come to me for treatment. If anyone starts asking loads of questions, seems to be fired up with curiosity and intrigued by the subconscious mind and LCH, then I suggest they read my book. Those curious souls are in the minority, though. Most people don't read it.

There's quite a lot to take in, so I don't explain everything all at once, but I need to make sure that I get enough information across in an accessible way in the consultation session so they have the best chance of making the decision that is right for them, the decision on whether to go ahead with treatment or not. Some of the other details can wait until session 2 or 3.

I start by finding out what they've sought out treatment for. I don't explain much until I've got a fairly clear idea of what it is that's bothering them and in what way they want things to improve.

Pat: *I could role-play for you if you like.*

Me: Ok, so how can I help you?

Pat: *I have a fear of feathers. I know they're not dangerous, but they make me want to run away. I can't bear to be in the room with them. I know it's irrational but my heart pounds, my hands sweat, I feel faint and nauseous and will get away from them if I possibly can.*

Me: Ok. That's enough for me to start my explanations. In a consultation, I'd be asking more questions but for this purpose, I don't need to know anything else for now.

You said, "I know it's irrational". That's a term that people often use for when something doesn't seem to make sense.

Let's just think about the mind for a moment. This fear of feathers exists in your mind but you don't want it. You find it uncomfortable and inconvenient and as far as you know, there's no risk of any kind of danger involved, but you can't get rid of the fear. No amount of reasoning or willpower will take it away. You didn't ever decide to create that fear. It just appeared one day or gradually developed over time.

To explain about LCH, I need you to think about the mind in very simple terms. Imagine it being composed of two parts, the conscious mind and the subconscious mind. It helps me to explain if you imagine the two parts are two people. You are the conscious mind and I'd like you to imagine there's another person on the chair next to you, and that person is your subconscious mind.

Pat: *That sounds a bit weird.*

Me: Humour me for now, please, and I'm sure you'll find it makes some kind of sense before long.

Pat: *Ok*

Me: You have this fear. You didn't create it, you don't want it and you don't know why it's there. Your thinking, reasoning, conscious mind, the part you are aware of and have some control over, didn't create this fear. The fear exists within you, so it must have been created by your subconscious mind. That's what irrational means, in my opinion. It's not exactly that it doesn't make sense. It's more that it makes no sense to the conscious mind. In my opinion, an irrational fear only exists because it makes perfect sense to the subconscious mind.

Pat: *I'm trying to imagine my subconscious. Is it a man or a woman?*

Me: I tend to think of mine as a woman. What do you think?

Pat   *Maybe it doesn't matter because we're only looking at it as if it were a person and it isn't really. Let's assume it's a man for now.*

Me: Ok. So there's no point in my working directly with you, on a conscious level, to resolve this fear of feathers. You don't know anything that can fix it because if you did, you would have fixed it for yourself, wouldn't you?

Pat: *Yes. This is costing me time and money. If I could have sorted it out myself, then I wouldn't have needed to come to you for help.*

Me: So I need to work with him, the guy on the chair next to you.

Pat: *How do you do that?*

Me: Imagine that you and he are good friends and he's the quiet one. You always do all the talking but in this case, he's the one who has all the information. I need to help you get so nicely relaxed that you can't be bothered to join in the conversation. He knows everything but he can't collaborate with me while you're chattering away.

Pat: *So how do you get me to shut up?*

Me: That's where the hypnosis comes in. It's a way of getting you into such a comfortable and relaxed state, both physically and mentally, that you can't be bothered to keep up with the conversation. You just want the world to leave you in peace to enjoy a pleasant day-dream from your comfy chair.

    Once you're in that state, I can work with your subconscious and help him to re-examine why he created this fear and see if any of the information he has is incorrect or out of date in any way. He's a conscientious guy, so he'll be happy to sort anything out that he discovers isn't totally accurate.

Pat: *How do you get me into that 'can't be bothered state'?*

Me: I need to get the chair that you're sitting in reclined, encourage you to get yourself comfortable, and then give some instructions and suggestions that, if you go along with me and let me guide you, then you'll find yourself getting gradually more and more relaxed.

    I also need to encourage your subconscious mind to help the process along. He's conscientious and he has your best interests at heart, so he needs to know, before we start, that you and he are in safe hands. I'm not going to ever tell him what to do, any more than I would switch off the smoke alarm just because the noise was irritating me. I'd switch off the toaster, the hob, the oven, or whatever it was that I'd left on. I'd get an electrician if there was an electrical fault. I'd make sure it was safe before I pressed the 'silence' button.

This fear of feathers, to me, is like the noise of the smoke alarm. It's telling us that something isn't right and needs our attention. Maybe there's some smoke, the beginnings of a fire or some other emergency.

The only instructions I give are to help you relax, and from then on, my work is focussed on collaborating with your subconscious to help him fully resolve this fear of feathers in a safe and thorough way.

Once your subconscious understands that, he is likely to help you relax so that each of you can play your own individual part in your treatment.

Pat: *What kinds of things can LCH be used for and be beneficial for?*

Me: Generally, things that don't seem to make sense to the conscious mind. For example, a fear of poisonous snakes is a rational fear. We wouldn't want to get rid of that fear. A fear of dangerous animals or situations helps to keep us safe. Your fear of feathers leaves you and me puzzled, so the subconscious mind must have created it. That means we can work with the subconscious to resolve it.

Something that affects most people, like a mild or moderate fear of exams or a driving test is unlikely to be one for which LCH would bring benefit. On the whole, it's again a quite useful reaction that keeps us on our toes. It usually makes us work harder and be more focussed.

We wouldn't expect to be able to remove a normal reaction to a severe life-experience, such as grief when a loved-one dies or nightmares and flashbacks soon after a traumatic experience.

If the sufferer believes the cause is external to them, that it's in their genes, that it's someone else's fault, if they are not prepared to consider that something inside of them is playing a part, then LCH might still be beneficial for whatever symptom they are suffering from, but they are unlikely to have the motivation or the understanding to play their part, so I wouldn't expect a positive outcome in such a situation.

Pat: *So the symptom needs to be one that fits with LCH and the client needs to play their part too?*

Me: That's right.

Pat: *Ok. That'll do for now.*

And in real life?

Chris: *You couldn't tell us about any of your clients before. Has anyone given you permission to tell their story now?*

Me: Yes. Four people have very kindly given me permission. Clearly I'm not going to give their real names and have agreed with them on what needs to be disguised to maintain their anonymity, but apart from that, these are true stories. It's an account of their treatments and the effects they have experienced as a result, some described in their own words but mainly in mine.

They've all got something specific about them, some aspect of their response to treatment that you might not expect. There are two men and two women. Two got a simple successful outcome where the symptom they were struggling to cope with simply went away. The other two had that kind of success but also got some bonuses, some wider benefits, some positive side-effects.

Two were completed in just a handful of sessions and the other two took at least 10 sessions.

Three of them came to me for a symptom that many people would expect could be successfully treated using hypnotherapy. The other one was totally different.

What do you expect is possible from working with the subconscious mind using hypnotherapy?

Pat: *I'd expect some changes in people's habits, reducing unwanted ones, maybe for a few months or for a few years and maybe needing a top-up from time to time.*

Chris: *I'd expect benefits for habits, phobias, anxiety, panic attacks, insomnia, that kind of thing, but nothing physical. If it's a physical symptom, then it needs a medical treatment. If the specialist says there's no cure yet, then maybe hypnotherapy could provide some help to live with it, manage it, until there's some medical and/or surgical intervention developed and tested and proved to be effective and safe.*

Me: Hmmm... so maybe the subconscious has some surprises in store for you. Maybe hypnotherapy has more to offer than you anticipate.

Maybe we can begin to open the door a little bit wider so we can take a longer look from a different perspective...

CHAPTER 2

If I could wave a magic wand what would 'happily ever after' look and feel like?

Pat: *Are you able to tell us some of those real-life stories right now?*

Me: Yes. I have permission from someone who came to me to lose weight, someone who had a gluten allergy, someone who wanted to give up smoking and someone who wanted to be rid of their habit of biting their nails.

Chris: *Tell us about the person who wanted to lose weight first. I've been watching programmes on the TV about how our modern lifestyle is playing a huge part in causing us to put on weight. The documentaries describe how the car, the washing machine, the countless labour-saving devices we use reduce the number of calories we burn. The food we eat is becoming more concentrated and calorie-rich so we eat more before we feel satisfied and full. How can you help people overcome the effects of the way most of us live our lives today?*

Me: I've seen some of those programmes too, and I agree that there's a lot in our environment that is pulling and pushing us in the direction of gaining more and more weight. Gaining that extra weight is, in turn, leading more and more of us towards related illnesses such as Type II diabetes and heart disease. But we have a huge resource of our own that is so powerful if the conscious and subconscious parts of our mind are pulling in the same direction. If they are working in tune and in time with each other like pairs of Olympic rowers, then we, as individuals, can find and follow the right path for ourselves, whatever, within reason, the world puts in our way.

Imagine a canoeist who has trained for many years and developed the skills, mental and physical, and the strength, again mental and physical, to navigate white water safely and efficiently. Our conscious and sub-conscious mind can and do work well together as a team. We've learnt to navigate an extremely complex and, in some parts, hostile world. We've learnt those skills by taking one small step at a time and learning a whole encyclopaedia full of lessons from each and every tiny step.

Pat: *Ok. I'll go with that for now. We can theorise forever, but it's really the results that matter. I'm intrigued to know how this person's treatment went.*

Let me introduce...

Me: Her name is Clare, and before she first came
to see me, if she wasn't dieting and just let
herself eat what she wanted, she would put on
a pound or two most weeks. The long term
effects of that, with the occasional brief attempt
at some new kind of diet, was that she gained
about 3 stone in 2 years.

She would eat a fairly standard diet of three
fairly healthy meals a day with maybe elevenses
and maybe supper, whatever else she needed to
keep herself going in the meantime.

Some of her extra off-diet routines included a
trip with a friend, every month or so, for a
meal out. Their choice would often be fish, chips
and peas, tea, bread and butter in a restaurant
famous for catering to the appetites of
connoisseurs of such a treat. Other favourites
were occasional visits to the coast, where tea or
coffee and cakes were traditional. Locally and
freshly caught fish meant that there was only one
logical choice from the cafe's main meal menu.
On a weekly basis, Saturday brunch included
grilled bacon and 2 poached eggs with toast.

During the periods when she tried to control
her eating, she would go on a specific diet or
she would simply change one aspect of her food
intake. She might choose to eat more fruit and
vegetables and less of the sweet, rich, snack-
food treats. She might do without some of her
off-diet habits. She would tend to manage this

fairly easily for a while but eventually, she would weaken from the mental effort of will it required from her. She would then give in to that strong sense of injustice that she was depriving herself of food and outings that others were happily savouring.

She would eat that apple or pear or plain salad as planned, but occasionally crave the chocolate biscuit or the bag of crisps. That craving wouldn't let her rest until she had fed it what it really wanted. Nothing else would satisfy that hungry gremlin inside her once it got an idea into its head.

She almost never really felt full while eating. She might feel over full and a bit sickly once the plate or bag or packet was empty, but not notice anything of how she felt while there was still food left in front of her. The one exception was at Christmas time, especially when there were guests to feed and entertain. When it seemed like they'd only just finished one meal and it was time to sit down to the next, when there was a food mountain that never seemed to get any smaller, it would take that kind of rare event to get her to that 'couldn't eat another mouthful' kind of fullness.

Off-diet, the feeling of physical hunger, of an empty and grumbling, rumbling stomach, was also unfamiliar to Clare, but that didn't seem to impact on her habit of wandering into the kitchen during an evening's relaxation in front of the TV. While the adverts were on, she would stand in front of the fridge or the cupboard thinking 'what can I have now?'

She had given up smoking about 12 years before she first contacted me. She had swapped those cigarettes, using nicotine replacement and a manageable degree of effort of will, for biscuits and other snacks, so that her morning coffee and afternoon tea felt complete without smoking.

It seemed like the lesser of two evils to go for something to eat rather than smoking and she assumed, at the time, that she would be able to sort out her diet once the nicotine was out of her system and those associations with lighting up were distant memories. But, 12 years on, she found herself still struggling with her weight.

She also retired around that time, which left her less active routinely, and she moved into a bungalow so she didn't climb stairs quite so often during an average day.

When dieting, she would check her progress once a week. She would be drawn automatically to those dreaded bathroom scales, to hold her breath as she waited for the reading and to hope for some sign that the previous week hadn't been that bad. She faced that every week, month after month, year after year, and was worn down by it all, seeing no end in sight to her wearying battle of will.

That full length mirror in the bedroom was dreaded like the bathroom scales. She tended not to look at herself because she hated what she saw. She was disgusted with the sight of herself and disappointed with herself for not being able to do anything about it.

As a young child, she remembered always having to clear her plate. She grew up in the 1940's and 50's when food was scarce and much more expensive in comparison to earnings than it is today. She would never have been allowed to leave anything then and carried that habit through a fair few decades. She was still carrying it when she first came to see me in 2011. She didn't think that habit would ever change.

She hated to waste food, and found it very difficult to let a plate go back to the kitchen when out for a restaurant meal, leaving anything to be scraped into the bin. The same was true when eating at home. From deep down inside her, it just felt so wrong.

What do we think?

Chris: *That sounds like a familiar picture for quite a lot of people.*

Pat: *Yes. If we don't identify with at least some of that personally, most, if not all, of us know someone, a close friend or colleague or relation, who lives that life.*

So what happened, then?

Me: I will tell you, but first I want to ask you a question.

    What would be your dream solution to this? If I could wave a magic wand, what would her 'happily ever after' look and feel like?

Chris: *I'd imagine her weighing much less, fitting into comfortably looser but also smaller sized clothes. She would be able to control her eating, keep her calorie intake down much more easily and stick to her diet long term.*

Pat: *I'd say the ideal would be a healthy but strict diet that would get her down to her target weight in just a few months, so she wouldn't get disillusioned, and then a healthy but not so strict diet that was easy to stick to and that maintained her new healthy weight. That's what seems to be the difficult aspect for most people. Once they stop being strict with themselves, they seem to go off in the other direction and end up putting the weight back on, even more than they had originally lost. She needs help to stop herself getting into that trap, I think.*

Me: Ok. Thanks for that. Now I'm going to paint a different kind of 'happily ever after' picture for you to consider.

    These new habits and effects start emerging steadily and automatically over a period of weeks or months: -

        Rather than eating food to stop it going to waste, putting it in the fridge for later that day or for the next day's lunch.

Noticing, during the meal, a feeling of the stomach beginning to be full enough, beginning to feel satisfied. A few mouthfuls later, putting down the cutlery without giving it a second thought, certainly without any internal debate or tug-of-war.

Noticing how much food is enough to create that lovely full-enough feeling and using that learning to amend how much is bought from the shops, how much is cooked and served up for each meal, what and how much is ordered when eating out.

Enjoying food and savouring each mouthful. Not wanting to miss that experience by eating absent-mindedly in front of the television.

No longer noticing any of the above as it happens but on reflection, when asked about it, being aware that those habits are still in place and that weight is steadily reducing.

Forgetting to get on the scales and, from time to time, getting something out of the back of the wardrobe and finding it fits again. Going shopping for clothes and picking out the usual size only to find that a smaller one would fit better.

Getting on with life without a constant preoccupation with food, eating and weight. Having more time and energy, physical and psychological, for aspects of life that had previously been squeezed out by an almost life-long diet/weight management battle.

In summary, turning into the dieting/weight equivalent of a life-long non-smoker rather than a continually struggling ex-smoker.

So what do you think of that as a 'happily ever after'?

Pat: *That would certainly fit a 'magic wand' kind of fairy story for me. It sounds too farfetched. I don't believe that ever really happens. Decades of habits don't just reverse themselves in a few weeks and months.*

Chris: *I agree and I'm not interested in fiction. Tell us what really happened.*

Me: That wasn't fiction. That was the truth, the facts, exactly as I've described. Clare has read and validated it.

Pat: *Ok, now I've got to know how you did that. Take me through it step by step.*

Me: Fine. I'll start by going through the sessions one by one.

CHAPTER 3

The two parts of the mind arrive at my door because they are at odds with each other

When she first emailed me for an appointment, Clare was keen to get some relief.

'...Because of my weight, depression is now becoming an issue so time for action!...'

Session 1

The consultation

Clare wanted to lose weight. She had explored every avenue she had ever heard of and had only had short-term success. Stepping back from a life of serial-dieting, of occasional successes, of battles fought and won, only to be defeated again soon afterwards, she wanted to put an end to the war. Her objective was to resolve it once and for all. She needed some help.

What she had tried so far

She had tried every diet/exercise regime going but it had always felt like such an uphill struggle. It would get her down and then she would eat and drink to ease the pain. Then she would get mad with herself and sink into a downward and depressing spiral.

She also suffered osteoarthritis, and this reduced her ability to exercise in the way she would like to. That had taken away one of the measures she had previously used to help herself lose weight. Those painful joints also gave her more reasons to turn to food for comfort, relief and distraction.

Her GP prescribed her some medication that is designed to prevent the body from absorbing the fat contained in her diet. Although it had some unpleasant side-effects which were exacerbated on days when she wasn't able to keep her fat intake to a minimum, it was a testament to her determination and strength of will that she persevered for 8 months. Her reward for all that effort was tiny. She experienced only a small and short-lived improvement.

Another medical intervention started with some routine tests that led to a diagnosis of an underactive thyroid. She had been on medication for many years and regular thyroid function tests every 12 months had shown that she was stable on the same level of that medication for the last 4 or 5 years. Her thyroid gland, her metabolism, was being pharmaceutically assisted to work at a healthy normal level.

She stopped smoking for financial and health reasons, and had achieved that with a combination of willpower and nicotine inhalers. It took her about 6 months to gain that 'non-smoker' feeling which is still with her today, about 12 years on.

She didn't often have cravings for specific foods and didn't have a particularly sweet tooth. She would absent-mindedly 'graze' while watching TV, or if bored, and would comfort-eat if she felt stressed.

How I could help

I'd got enough of a picture about what she wanted help with so it was time for me to tell her about what I had to offer. I explained a little about the subconscious mind, about LCH and some of the theory behind it.

We would need to work together with the aim of digging up some mental weeds – the habits she had never intended to plant in the first place. Some of the measures she had tried so far had felt like pulling and tugging unsuccessfully at those unwanted eating habits, that unsightly greenery in her virtual garden. She occasionally gained temporary relief by simply chopping the tops off – some new diet worked well for a while, the weight came off but then piled back on. With LCH, we get right to the roots and dislodge them so they come away quite easily.

If chopping the tops off is all we do, then we might be strengthening those unwanted and hardy plants just like we do when we prune the roses. To get rid of the weeds for good, we need to dig down until we've loosened them at the roots and carefully removed all traces so there's nothing left to grow back.

I believe we are meant to be happy and healthy and that, when we encounter an obstacle to that, the measures we put in place should lead to improvements. If that's not happening, then I believe there's likely to be some kind of misunderstanding in the way, just like there usually is when two close friends fall out with each other. Such a misunderstanding plants a seed that then germinates, grows roots and develops into weeds that strangle the beautiful scented plants we chose and planted and nurtured in the first place.

Clare could see that her attempts, up to then, had been targeted mainly at the surface. It made sense of her experience of losing weight temporarily and then gaining back even more than she had lost. She had been following diets that worked by pruning the weeds.

LCH teases out such misunderstandings and helps them to be re-examined and then understood more accurately. The two close friends who fell out, in this case, are the two parts of the mind. The conscious part is unhappy about something the subconscious part has put in place, like eating habits and weight in Clare's case, and they are unable to resolve it for themselves. They are like a couple who need relationship counselling because one of them wants to talk and analyse and fix their 'problem' and the other doesn't. Maybe the other one doesn't want to talk or finds themselves unable to. Maybe the quiet one doesn't see the issue as a problem at all and doesn't feel the need to make any changes.

LCH could be seen as a form of relationship counselling that works by finding what is really getting in the way.

Unlike the way a biased friend of one of them might aim to persuade the other partner to change the unwanted habit, the therapist starts from a position of assuming both are doing their best and have the best of intentions.

The couple started their relationship in harmony and agreement with each other but at some point on that journey, one of them unintentionally, inadvertently, accidentally, stepped off that happy, healthy path onto one that was unhappy, unhealthy, unsafe.

Because the one who took that step away did so without noticing what they'd done and where they had ended up as a result, they need help to retrace their steps and find that point at which they took that tiny step in that unhealthy direction.

Just as, with any relationship that is foundering (filling with water and then sinking) or floundering(struggling or moving with difficulty as in mud), something needs to change. Habitual ways of communicating are not working well enough for this deeper work to be facilitated.

We need to work more directly with the subconscious mind, the quiet one, and there are various measures that need to be put in place in the early stages of treatment. We help the subconscious step forward and join in and help the conscious mind relax and let their back-room assistant show their skills and complete whatever restorative work emerges as a result.

Her previous experience of hypnotherapy

Clare had had a prior experience of hypnosis, to stop smoking, but it hadn't gone well. It was about 20 years before. She had gone with a group of friends, 5 of them in all, to someone who described himself as a hypnotist. He treated them one at a time – great! - but they were all in the same room throughout the proceedings – hmmm....

As each one was being given the suggestions needed to induce hypnosis and then the instructions needed to remove cravings, urges, habits of smoking, the rest were watching and giggling. It didn't go well. She described it as a farce. The first thing they all did on leaving his office was to light up.

When people tell me about previous unproductive experiences they've had, I'm always so relieved that they are prepared to see it as a one-off and not indicative of hypnotherapy as a whole. Maybe they wonder if the therapist they saw wasn't right for them. Maybe they understand or at least consider that there are various types of hypnotherapy and that they haven't yet found the one that meets their own specific, individual needs.

In Clare's case, the person she had seen described himself as a hypnotist and she regarded that as something completely different from a hypnotherapist. I'm so glad she did.

A diagnosis, a syndrome or a specific, focussed target

I have a small amount of medical information gained
in a professional capacity several decades ago when
I qualified and worked as a psychiatric nurse. My
interpretations may not be totally up to date, things
may well have changed substantially since then – the
1980's - but I'll just continue to tell it as well as I can
and hope to be advised of any inaccuracies so that
I can amend or correct as appropriate.

My understanding of the traditional medical model is
that it starts with recording any relevant signs and
symptoms. A symptom is something we experience, we
notice, we suffer, like a pain or a rash or an unwanted
habit. A sign is something that is observed or detected,
maybe from a test, like a raised blood-pressure or some
chemical component of a urine or blood sample that is
outside of normal range.

A particular diagnosis is made based on the presence of
some or all of a specific set of these signs and symptoms
and once a diagnosis is achieved, then evidence-based
research dictates the best treatment regime.

LCH works from a different perspective. We don't infer
any connection between signs and symptoms in one
person based on there being a proven connection for
some or even many other people and we focus directly
on one symptom at a time.

People normally come to see us for help with an
unwelcome symptom.

We wouldn't normally be asked by clients to focus on signs.

If they have a worrying sign detected by some routine medical testing or screening, then it might also be something that LCH could bring some benefit for. That's more or less what happened to me in the treatment I received, described in some detail in 'What if it really is... ?'

People, in general, would probably not currently consider this kind of treatment for signs detected by various kinds of tests and screening. In the future though, as LCH grows and develops, as more and more therapists deliver unexpected benefits, positive side effects, maybe more people will look at this complementary therapy as another productive resource for physical health as well as peace of mind.

All we can work with is what is affecting our client, what is bothering them, what they want to change or fix or get rid of.

Clare described various aspects of what could be described as a syndrome, relating to food, her eating habits, her weight and her size. We needed to agree which was the aspect she wanted to change, and if more than one, we needed to determine which one was at the top of her wish-list.

If she could carry on eating as she did but be at the weight she wanted, then she would be very happy.

Her eating habits were really only bothering her because of the effects they were having on her weight.

Many of us know, or know of, people who eat tiny amounts on a daily basis and still carry excess weight. Equally, there are people who eat far more than the healthy guideline amounts and don't appear to gain any extra body fat.

Some of the latter have been given medical tests such as MRI scans which have led to them being described as TOFIs. It stands for 'Thin on the Outside, Fat on the Inside'. They carry large amounts of visceral fat. This is the fat that surrounds internal organs, and we all need some of that kind of fat. Large quantities of it, though, are believed to be far more dangerous to our health than the subcutaneous fat that is clearly visible on the surface.

Equally, some people never feel full. Their life is totally disrupted because of a constant need to eat, all day long. Whether their weight is affected or not, their first wish is to achieve that satisfying feeling after a meal so they can get on with their lives and their work and play for at least a few hours before they need to eat again.

For these kinds of reasons, some people want their eating habits to change first. Their weight is of secondary importance to them.

Many people believe that the relationship between food, exercise, body-weight and body-fat isn't quite as simple as that familiar message implies – eat more calories than you use up and you'll gain weight – eat fewer than you use and you'll lose weight. The metabolic rate is part of the formula, and that rate can change over time.

Repeated dieting can cause a reaction within the body, turning down the rate at which the food is processed. I believe that the subconscious mind can and does play a part in turning the boiler thermostat up or down, too. That's part of why, when working with the subconscious, it feels so important to separate out the two aspects of the issue, eating and weight, focus attention on them one at a time and make sure both are fully resolved.

If we achieve a change in the eating habits and fewer calories are taken in, but we haven't resolved the need for a certain level of weight or a certain body size or shape, then a compensating reduction in the metabolic rate can prevent the desired and expected weight loss.

For Clare, the eating was a secondary concern. She wanted to lose weight to help with some of the physical effects of the extra that she was carrying, such as the strain on her joints, in particular, a painful knee that didn't seem to be recovering properly. We agreed to initially target her difficulty or inability to lose weight and she wanted to lose 2 stone.

The decision to go ahead

It's important to make sure we have exchanged all the relevant information before we each make our decision on whether to proceed. I was satisfied that what she described was a symptom that LCH would be appropriate for and that the way she had responded to my explanations showed she had both understood it all and agreed with me, so was likely to also respond well to treatment.

I asked if she wanted to go ahead and she didn't show any signs of hesitation. She had made up her mind. It wasn't until much later that we talked about her first impressions and what helped her to decide.

The decision hadn't happened just at the point when I had asked her. She had begun to decide a few days earlier.

Clare was sceptical at first because she didn't see how hypnotherapy could help her, but she had tried everything else with no long-term success so it seemed worth at least enquiring further. She had contacted another therapist and been informed that she would need to pay for a number of sessions up front, before treatment could begin, before even meeting the therapist. There was no guarantee of success on offer and no refund available if it didn't work or treatment wasn't right for her. She didn't like the sound of that arrangement.

I have a different policy. She learnt from my website that she was under no obligation. She would be able to discuss her needs with me and learn more about what I had to offer, and then she could make up her mind. She would only start to pay if she decided to go ahead with treatment, and she would pay for each session on the day, not paying for a course of sessions in advance.

Some people ask how many sessions it will take to complete treatment, and others understand from my explanations about the problem-solving nature of LCH that it's impossible to predict exactly. It's important for people to understand what to expect especially when time and money are scarce resources, which they are for most of us, for most of our lives.

We sometimes need a quick fix for something that is of little importance to us. If a plastic food box we bought from a discount shop fell apart after a year, we would simply throw it away and buy another. On the other hand, we would take the trouble to take a TV back to the shop if it broke down after a month.

If something is bothering us, and bothering us a lot, and bothering us most of the time, then most of us would see it as time and money well spent to get it fully resolved rather than putting a sticking plaster over it and ignoring it until the plaster fell off.

We had that kind of discussion to help Clare take all the relevant information into account and she decided to go ahead because it was something she really wanted to fix and she felt quite inspired by my explanations. She remembered thinking 'What have I got to lose?'

The first experience of hypnosis

Technically, it wasn't her first experience of hypnosis that day, but whether or not she had really entered into a properly relaxed state on that previous anti-smoking treatment, I needed to help her benefit and enjoy it much more this time.

As her session with the hypnotist had been one she hadn't fully engaged with, and I can't imagine many people would under those circumstances, it was important to explain what she could expect and how she could play her part.

The consultation takes place while the client is sitting in a reclining chair in its upright position. The next step involves the chair being moved into its reclined position where, like a sun-lounger, it goes into an almost horizontal comfortably supportive curviness. I talk to the client and guide them gradually into a more relaxed state. The client needs to know what to expect so they feel safe to allow me to guide them in that way.

When we lie in bed on a day off, or on a lazy, chilled-out holiday, the bed comfy and cosy, and with no specific time we need to get up by, we can consider getting up – and we will – in a while. If the phone rings or someone knocks at the door, we can decide that they'll leave a message or they'll come back later, and turn over to rest and enjoy that comfort a bit longer.

If the phone rings repeatedly, or if someone hammers on the door, then we'll know that it's probably urgent and we'll get up and deal with it.

So, in the same way, with hypnosis, we know what's going on, we can tell if something needs doing, but most of the time, if it can wait, then we'll let it. We just can't be bothered and we're too comfortable to move if we don't have to.

Some people have understandable fears of an unknown, unfamiliar mental state. Some have seen stage hypnosis, heard words like 'trance' and 'out of control' and need reassurance that nothing like that will happen to them.

There are some swimming pools, mainly in the grounds of hotels in sun-drenched holiday resorts, where there is a gentle walkway into the water, with no sudden drops. If we're a bit unsure, a bit nervous, for some reason, we can walk along, holding on to the rail, dip our toes in the pleasantly warm blueness that gently massages our feet and ankles as we take one small step after another.

We can decide, when it reaches our ankles or our calves, that that's far enough for today, stay there and enjoy that for awhile before turning round and walking back out. The next day, we walk confidently to where we left off the day before. From there, we take a few more steps until the water is up to our knees. By the end of the week, we've gone deep enough to swim a few strokes.

The client might have no idea what to expect from hypnosis. They might fear a leap into the unknown, like jumping off the diving board into a pool of unknown depth filled with water of unknown temperature.
The first experience of hypnosis is like that first gentle dipping of toes into warm and shallow water, with no expectation or pressure to go any deeper than feels right and comfortable.

As part of the way the client plays their own part in the treatment, they are asked to take a CD home with them at the end of that session and practise relaxing to that CD about once a day between the sessions. This is how they gradually relax more and more, maybe going deeper and deeper into that 'can't be bothered' feeling where the conscious mind is off duty and the subconscious mind has time and space to play its own vital part in the process.

Each CD lasts about 20 minutes and is simply a recording of me talking in a similar way to the hypnosis session experienced with me in person. It's not one of those CDs to fall asleep to, so for most people, it's usually best to avoid listening last thing at night.

By the time they come back for session 2, clients tend to have reached that point where they're 'deep enough to swim', ready for the process of treatment to begin. Hypnosis, in LCH treatment, is very much like that gentle introduction to the pool. On the very first experience, in session 1, the client will go as far as is right for them. It may be the calves or the ankles or the knees or beyond. There is no right or wrong, no good or bad, no expectation to live up to. There is just the place that is right for that individual person and whatever state they arrived in on that very first day.

All of that information about when and how to practise is on the 'CD Guidelines' leaflet that accompanies the CD. I explain all of that in the first session, but there is so much to absorb at that time that it helps to have a reminder of the key points before playing the CD at home.

But the client also needs to understand why as well as when and how to practise. In the relaxed state that develops more and more with each practice, the conscious mind is beginning to drift off more quickly and more easily and become more of a passenger in the car being driven by the subconscious. The conscious mind gets more and more used to looking out of the window at the view as the subconscious decides where to take them both. The subconscious mind gets more and more used to deciding where to go, what to see, without the conscious mind 'helping' or taking over.

As a result, the two parts of the mind settle in more easily each session into their respective roles that facilitate the subconscious mind working more directly with me towards re-examining and reassessing long-forgotten subconscious information. The first experience of hypnosis and the CD practice between sessions 1 and 2 are the first steps towards a new way of communicating that's needed to resolve a previously intractable dilemma.

Clare was happy to put her feet up and enjoy her first experience of relaxing to my voice. Although it lasted 25 minutes, it felt more like 10 minutes to her, which was a clue to both of us that she had been even more relaxed than she had realised. She hadn't been asleep, but her perception of the passage of time had been much more random and incorrect, like it is during sleep, than the accuracy most of us enjoy when we're wide awake.

She had relaxed more deeply than she had expected to, and in general, was happy with how it had gone. She left with a new and unfamiliar feeling. Up to then, she had always felt as if she was on her own. That had changed. She knew she didn't need to fight that battle alone any more. Someone was helping her and she enjoyed a refreshing sense of relief that she was in a place where someone understood. This might actually work for her!

Session 2 – one week later

Her CD practice had been a bit mixed. On occasions, she had fallen asleep. A few people experience that, and, as I need my clients to be nicely relaxed but awake during sessions, my advice to anyone who does is to arrange a slightly more upright position for themselves. Lying on the bed or the settee, with just one pillow or cushion, will often be all it takes for my voice to guide the listener into slumber. Practising at a different time of day helps some people too.

Many of us experience that lovely 'drifting off to sleep' experience to the sound of the TV or the radio, too, and it's exactly the same kind of sleep when it happens with the CD. It's quite natural, and there's no problem if that happens, except that it isn't helping with the response to treatment, so we need to reduce the tendency for that drifting off to sleep to happen.

Clare had practised with the CD 6 times, and on the occasions that she was awake and aware, she found that she noticed different parts of the recording each time. From the 'CD Practice Guidelines' leaflet that I'd given her, and discussed with her in Session 1, she knew that that was exactly what I was expecting. It was a good indicator that she, her conscious and her subconscious mind, and the CD were all doing their job in getting her ready to respond well to treatment.

Having played it 3 times and stayed awake right through, she had heard something on the second and third time that she had missed the times before. At times, her conscious mind, her attention, must have been wandering off, her imagination taking in the sights and sounds of maybe wandering along some fictional or remembered sunny beach or path through a forest.

That's a development that helps with the progress of treatment. It's part of how the conscious mind mentally goes off to relax with a good book so I can work with the subconscious mind with fewer curious interruptions and fewer 'helpful' interventions.

LCH treatment is underpinned by a process of working as directly as possible with the subconscious mind because we believe it's that part of the mind which created the consciously-unwanted symptom.

The two parts of the mind arrive at my door because they are at odds with each other and need some external help to remove any barriers to a life of harmony and collaboration.

Clare came back for session 2 with a mixture of feelings. She was excited as it looked to her as if she

might actually be going in the right direction at last.
At the same time, she was scared that she might be
putting too much hope and trust in her treatment, in
my ability to deliver it and her ability to respond to it.

I gave her some examples of the kind of responses
I've had from people with similar food / eating / weight
struggles.

Someone had noticed that, after eating a crisp from
her partner's packet, she had then not felt any urge to
go into the kitchen for a bag for herself – a first!

Someone had taken a bite from a piece of birthday
cake at a party and, an hour or so later, noticed that
the rest of that slice was still there on the plate in front
of her. She hadn't absent-mindedly nibbled her way
through the rest – unheard of, for her, up to then!

Others had gone out for a special meal, a birthday,
an anniversary, a last night of the holiday, and hadn't
fancied a pudding. They had felt happy with what
they'd eaten, had enjoyed the occasion, and gone
straight on to the coffee – on reflection, a big surprise!

She gained confidence in LCH and in my ability, but
then continued to question her own. Would it work
for her? Would she be able to respond in the way that
was needed?

Many people have those kinds of concerns, and it's often
very much a part of what they want to have treatment
for. Many have a niggling idea in the back of their mind

that wonders 'Am I good enough, clever enough, determined enough and maybe even, do I deserve this?'

My response to that was something like, "You can worry if you want to, and you possibly will until we've fixed the underlying cause, but I've seen enough to know that you have all you need within you already to respond to and benefit from the treatment you're receiving."

She described feeling somewhat reassured and certainly prepared to give herself the benefit of the doubt.

The first part of the process sometimes results in a memory coming to mind.

This happened for Clare. What she found herself remembering was from the age of 4, when her mother was just about to give birth to her younger sister. Clare had been sent to stay with her grandma. That might have been fairly sad for her, but it had an added puzzling and painful twist. Her younger brother, then aged 2, stayed with Mum and Dad. She didn't know why she had been the only one they had 'sent away' at the time.

If the memory that comes to mind is one that the client has long regarded as being 'the cause' or at least, a powerful nudge in the direction of the symptom or issue we are treating, then it's likely to be mainly conscious-mind-generated information.

If we get a familiar memory, but one that has never been thought of as relevant in any way to the symptom, as happened to Clare during that session, or if we get just an image that doesn't trigger any kind of remembered association at all, then the conscious mind is unlikely to have played any part in generating it.

If everything in the mind is either conscious or subconscious, because we've defined the subconscious as the residual, everything that isn't conscious, then the image must have been mainly subconsciously generated.

People often find that this session is the only one that triggers memories for them, information coming back to them, to their conscious mind. That's because, as treatment progresses, we are able to use more sophisticated techniques that allow the conscious mind to drift further and further away from the process of treatment.

The CD practice also helps that distancing to develop more and more. Many people find it empowering to be given a simple and practical way for them to help their treatment become more efficient and effective.

Instead of standing at the viewing bay watching the mechanic service and MOT the car, we are guided to the hospitality suite where there's a coffee machine and a DVD player with loads of our favourite films on the shelf to choose from. As this kind of experience is repeated at home with each time the CD is played, an automatic response begins to develop. The sound of my voice encourages a stronger and stronger feeling that this is 'time-off' for the conscious mind. That response becomes more and more valuable to the process of treatment as those more sophisticated techniques are introduced in later sessions.

When people do get memories, some are concerned and wonder what the information means. In such cases, I need to explain something about the significance of the stage of treatment we've reached at that point.

Imagine coming back from a memorable holiday in a beautiful resort on the Canary Island of Lanzarote. Your best friend wants to know all about it and quizzes you for every tiny detail. Neither of you has any interest in the journey, but, in order to get there, you took a taxi from your home to the station. Then you took a train to the airport followed by a flight and a coach journey.

Whether you took a taxi and train or drove to the airport or got a lift or whatever, is of no interest to either of you as you tell your story. You are both focussing on the final destination, the chilling by the pool with a good book, the delicious local food and drink, the sight-seeing, the night-life and so on.

But in order to get to Lanzarote and have those experiences, you had to undertake a journey that had at least 3 legs to it, the transfer to the home airport, the flight, the transfer to the resort. It doesn't matter precisely which method or route you took for the first leg of the journey. All that matters is that, for the second leg of the journey to take place, the first leg has to have already been completed.

In treatment, we are on the trail of the final destination, the underlying cause. Equally, in treatment, we are on a journey of at least 3 legs. What we focus on in session 2 is completing the first leg of the journey. Once completed, we can start the second leg of the journey in session 3.

Once we're on the flight, we've forgotten about the journey from home to airport. We're looking forwards in the journey, not back.

In the same way, session 2 concludes when we reach the home airport, so we don't need to spend any further time, in or between treatment sessions, focussing on leg 1 of the journey.

One important aim of session 2 is to help the conscious mind take a step back in the proceedings and to encourage the subconscious mind to step forward. From that forward position, the subconscious can then help guide the journey to find the hidden treasure and unlock the secret which has been maintaining a constant frustrating battle between the two parts of the mind.

Clare took that first leg of the journey effectively and was relieved to learn that she didn't need any more of that kind of memory. She was also happy to find that she wasn't required to play much of a part consciously in her treatment. She didn't need to analyse. She didn't need to try.

We agreed that her job, at this stage, was to play the CD once a day and just let her eating pattern adjust and settle itself without using any amount of willpower or doing any kind of dieting.

Session 3 – one week later

She found the CD practice a bit more of a challenge that time. She had worked out what was needed from her, and had been trying hard to achieve it. She so much wanted this to work that she was putting all her willpower into it. Unfortunately, trying and relaxing are at opposite ends of the spectrum, so we needed to find a way for her to allow the process to develop naturally rather than for her to strive to make it happen.

She found the techniques of session 3 worked well for her and we successfully progressed even further in the direction of greater subconscious involvement in the process and less activity from the conscious mind.

The techniques used from session 4 onwards work best when we're in that 'glazed eyes watching our partner's choice of TV program' kind of state. Some of us find our thoughts take us here and there and amuse or entertain us, or worry us, or irritate us in that free-form journey. We can learn to take hold of the steering wheel, or the map, or the TV remote of our inner entertainment media.

Clare chose to create mental pre-holiday shopping and packing lists, something she often does when her husband is watching the football. We'd found something that worked for her. She chose to create and update those lists as an effective way to keep her conscious mind occupied. She clearly understood what was needed from her. She had discovered a natural and easy way she could do her job of 'getting out of the way' which would enable and encourage her subconscious mind to get on with its own job of analysing and problem-solving in collaboration with me.

Session 4 – one week later

One way of looking at the work done in sessions 1 to 3 is to consider it as building foundations. Unless people understand that, they can feel puzzled and disappointed. They might even decide treatment isn't working, if they see and feel no improvement.

Firstly, imagine running something on the computer, like installing some new software or an upgrade to the BBC I-Player. Often, there's no indication, before you start, of the amount of time it's likely to take. If there's a progress bar that seems to be moving steadily towards its end point, then we can decide to sit and wait and enjoy a few moments of peace and quiet and the restful view from the window. If it seems to be progressing much more slowly than that, we might put the kettle on or even go for an early lunch.

Without that progress bar, we just don't know what to do. It might even have stopped or stalled and need re-starting. It might be broken and never finish however long we wait.

If the process of treatment is slightly more transparent, then clients can see how things are going and manage their own expectations, plan their finances, review and update their interim symptom-management strategies.

Back to the house-building analogy – building foundations. There's very little to see of the desired end-product, the house itself, for quite some time. The foundations are dug and filled with strong and stable materials around all the necessary pipes and cables, plumbing and drainage structures. A team of cowboys could throw up some walls and doors and windows and a roof quite quickly, and we might be impressed – until we moved in and found that the sinks and the bath didn't empty, the loo didn't flush and the lights and sockets didn't work.

It's because we know all this that we don't expect to see progress straight away when our dream house is being built.

If we understand that LCH is designed to be as strong, as functional and durable and as safe as houses, and because of that, it takes time to build the foundations, then we can have confidence that all is going well.

There seems to be a fairly widely held expectation that certain types of talking therapies such as psychotherapy take many months or years to complete, and that hypnotherapy takes a small number of sessions, sometimes just 1!

LCH sits somewhere between those two models in terms of how many sessions are needed for success, deep-rooted solutions, long term and substantial benefit without the need for maintenance or regular top-ups.

Clare had found my website from the internet and had nothing more to go on than the explanations it contained. She doesn't want other people to need that leap of faith she needed to keep her going. She wants people to read her story and see just what is possible with Lesserian™ Curative Hypnotherapy.

We had the foundations securely built and in session 4, we found something that needed another look. Something long-forgotten, from her childhood, had been one of those 'you should know better' moments that I'm sure all of us experienced when we were quite young. The signs seemed to indicate that her subconscious reassessed it, there and then, and then continued that process by readjusting the knock-on effects of the initial assessment. That processing will have been going on in the background, as she slept, as she watched TV, as she continued her day to day life, just like the way the computer does its security scanning as we type an email or watch a video clip on YouTube.

Session 5 – two weeks later

The signs that indicated a lot of constructive work had been going on came out of our discussion at the beginning of her next session. She had been exercising regularly for 3 weeks but hadn't yet lost any weight. Earlier that week, though, she had been eating a meal and hadn't cleared her plate. She hadn't noticed at the time, but she suddenly remembered that fact as we were catching up.

If we consider that she had cleared her plate, almost religiously, every meal, since it had been drummed into her as a youngster, then we might also consider that this is certainly something worth noting.

Suddenly, one day, quite a few decades later, she hadn't cleared her plate and she hadn't even noticed at the time. That means that there can't have been any willpower involved. She hadn't been trying to eat less or to break that plate-clearing habit. Her subconscious had made a change, and just like when some kind person did some maintenance for us while we were out - our computer runs a bit quicker, or that door doesn't stick any more - if we're busy getting on with our work, we might not even spot the difference at the time.

She'd had a small packet of biscuits, the kind you get with the complementary tea and coffee in a hotel, and had eaten one biscuit from the pack. She had put the rest in her handbag, and they were still there, several days later.

In that gap between sessions 4 and 5, she had turned down a trip for lunch at the fish and chip restaurant, something that she normally really enjoys. She just hadn't fancied it that day. She noticed, again on reflection, that she hadn't been turning to food quite so often in times of stress, and all of these developments were pretty well unheard of for her prior to session 4.

There were some fairly strong signs that something was readjusting deep within her subconscious mind.

She was very happy with those changes but was understandably cautiously watching and waiting and preparing herself, bracing herself in case it had been a misleadingly encouraging temporary blip.

We did some more work and her subconscious reassessed another childhood event and its repercussions.

Session 6 – 3 weeks later

Since the previous session, she'd had one of those occasional trips to the coast. She'd eaten three-quarters of the fish, half of the chips, none of the bread and butter. There were other examples of her feeling full and turning down extras because she didn't fancy them, including some of those famous continental chocolates. She'd been exercising, walking, swimming and gardening but she still hadn't lost any weight. Her clothes didn't feel any looser either but there was a slight feeling of her body being just a bit more firm and toned.

She came to see me about 3pm that day. It had got to 2pm and she had started to think about what else she needed to do before she set off. That was when she noticed feeling a bit hungry. She had had nothing to eat since breakfast at 7:30am and again, hadn't even noticed until afterwards. That feeling of hunger was a new and refreshingly reassuring one for her. In the past, if she wasn't dieting, then she wasn't ever hungry.

She had initially worried that she wouldn't be able to respond to treatment or that it wouldn't work for her, and although she had yet to lose any weight at all, she had seen so many signs of progress in her eating patterns and felt sure that it was only a matter of time.

The work done in this session seemed to be a process of joining a few stray dots left behind by some previous background processing. At this stage, it seemed possible that we had found all the roots already, which would mean that all the benefits she wanted were already in the pipeline - or there could be some remaining work to do.

We agreed that, once her subconscious stopped providing any more information to be reassessed, we would keep open a line of communication. She would ring me monthly and we would agree whether another session was needed based on how the month had gone. If she was finding it difficult, if she was having to make an effort to maintain those new eating patterns, then we would resume treatment and work on the sticking point.

She was very happy with that plan. She wasn't ready to let go of the lifeline yet. She hadn't made any progress towards her target weight and hadn't yet got confidence that these new habits and tendencies were here to stay.

Session 7 – six weeks later

Since session 6, she had been away on holiday. Just like in a previous session, it was only when we started to discuss the past few weeks that she noticed that she had left food on her plate at many of the meals while she was away. From her experience of previous similar holidays, she would have expected to have gained about 5lbs. In fact, she gained only 2 or 3 lbs. She had started going down from two poached eggs to one, and from a whole jacket potato to half of one.

On their own, they weren't enough to get excited about, but added to the other changes over the previous weeks, they seemed to be steady and consistent steps in the right direction.

We found yet another incident that her subconscious was ready to reassess and to reprocess, probably as thoroughly as it seems to have done with the others unearthed so far.

Session 8 – five weeks later

We both had to hold firm to our patience and belief in the good signs we'd seen so far, because, in spite of those new eating habits, smaller portions, stopping when full, and swimming twice a week, she actually gained a couple of lbs since session 7. Oh dear!

We continued our work. It seemed like what emerged from the session was just an observation of 'work in progress'. The subconscious seemed to be busy and we both just had to be patient and trust that it would complete all in good time.

Session 9 – four weeks later

Our patience was rewarded. She had lost 3lb and, not surprisingly, she was feeling more positive. It seemed like those new eating patterns were becoming more and more deep-rooted. She became more confident that they would continue. On top of the first real weight loss and the continued improvements in her eating patterns and her general sense of happiness, she was beginning to see improvements in her sleep.

She hadn't mentioned having any sleep problems up to that point, so I didn't even know about them, so of course, I hadn't treated them. Apparently, she had had great difficulty getting back off to sleep if she was ever disturbed in the night. She would normally lie awake for ages if anything woke her up in the early hours. More recently, she found that that had changed. She found herself going back off to sleep quite quickly and enjoying a good night's sleep in spite of any night-time noises outside.

Treatment that day was more of a tidying up exercise, mopping up the after-effects of work already completed and identifying the remaining few tasks still to be finalised.

Session 10 – one month later

Another strange and puzzling development had taken place since session 9. She found herself drawn much more to fish than meat. She had always routinely eaten fish once a week, but in recent weeks, was choosing it 3 or 4 times a week. Her sleep continued to be much better and her portion sizes continued to be smaller than before treatment began.

She had lost a few lbs before Christmas, and had put them back on over Christmas, but with her growing sense of optimism, she noticed that she would have normally put on quite a bit more annual festive weight than she had that year.

We had yet another treatment session that looked like more tidying up of loose ends. That time it seemed like all the roots had been dug up, but as always, we would have to wait and see.

And beyond

There haven't yet, to date, been any more treatment sessions. We spoke on the phone and she gave me an update on progress about once a month for about six months. The latest treatment session, session 10, was in January 2012.

In February, she reported having lost all the weight she had gained over Christmas, and that was in spite of having an injury that required her to put her feet up and rest for some significant period of time. She described feeling totally different about food now, always looking for the healthier options now, "*which is fantastic*!" She has had to start wearing a belt with her trousers as they were beginning to feel loose.

In March, the update still included being drawn to fish more than to meat, but also finding herself less drawn to carbohydrates. The weight loss was beginning to be more regular. She lost about 0.5lb a week, and was satisfied with that. As it was happening effortlessly, then she knew it was likely to be sustainable. She wasn't running on willpower. She was eating what she wanted, when she wanted, and her weight was going in the right direction. Happy days!

April was another productive month. She had lost 3.5lbs.

In early May, we saw a reduction in focus on exactly how much she had lost. It was 2 or 3 lbs. Maybe there was less need to monitor it quite so precisely. She was possibly spending that time and energy getting on with her life instead of needing to be so vigilant, as she had when she had been dieting. She had lost about 10lbs since the weight started to reduce between sessions 9 and 10.

By the end of May, she had gone past a stone in weight loss and was so happy with the results of her treatment that I asked how she would feel about people reading her story in my second book. She was happy to come and see me and allow me to interview her, so she could tell me her thoughts and reactions and I could paint this verbal picture.

She said, "*If it would help someone else, then I'd be happy to!*"

I say "Lovely generous lady!"

Chapter 4

Decades of habits reverse themselves in a few weeks and months

Swapping one symptom for another

Me: About 10 to 12 years before, Clare had given up smoking using will-power. She had turned her back on cigarettes and replaced them with rich, sweet snacks. Her weight had been fine prior to stopping smoking.

She had initially felt ok about the situation, because she presumed she would be able to go on a diet and all would then be fine. She didn't succeed. It didn't work.

Pat: *Did she swap one addiction for another?*

Me: I believe that that is highly likely to have been what happened. From the way I look at the subconscious and the way it works, it makes sense to me that the subconscious would let go of the smoking or the extra eating if we put some effort in. It seems likely that it wouldn't release its hold on both habits until the underlying cause, the roots, were fully resolved.

To date, no other unwelcome or unhealthy habits have crept in as her eating habits improved.

Habits and Addictions

Pat: *It seems to me that you use the terms habit and addiction interchangeably, but are they different, and if so, in what way?*

Me: There are several factors relevant for me here. One is that I aim to use the term the client uses. That's what they refer to it as. They might not be comfortable with the other term because, for example, addiction might seem too severe to relate to their level of irritation/frustration or habit might seem to trivialise the cause or nature of their intense suffering.

The term 'habit' seems neutral, in that we refer to good habits like cleaning our teeth, bad habits like putting loads of salt on our food, and just habits, like drinking tea or coffee in the morning.

By contrast, the term 'addiction' seems to imply judgement. We seem to need to explicitly specify 'positive addiction'. I don't think I've ever heard anyone refer to a 'negative addiction'. It sounds tautological.

I prefer the neutrality of using 'habit' where possible when speaking to clients in order to encourage the subconscious mind to collaborate with me. My aim is to help resolve the issue in whatever way is best for the client as a whole, their conscious and subconscious mind. I don't want to risk sending the message that I have pre-judged the situation and have taken sides.

Otherwise, habit and addiction seem to me to be almost synonyms and I can summarise the results of an internet search on that question: -

Habits develop from a conscious choice to do the same action or activity repeatedly. It gradually changes into something done automatically. At some point, if we decide we want to change or get rid of that action, it might take a little while and a bit of effort, but if it is purely a habit, we'll eventually succeed.

If we find we're stuck, if we can't make that change, if we try and succeed, at least for a while, and then suffer adverse reactions, from withdrawal symptoms, we probably need help. These activities or tendencies have progressed from habits into addictions. We can change a habit using willpower and other strategies but we usually need help to remove an addiction.

Sometimes, though, one of those terms just sounds wrong. I would struggle to refer to Clare's 'addiction to clearing her plate' even though it was an action she hadn't managed to change over many decades of trying.

Pat: *Ok. That makes sense of your interchangeable use.*

The placebo effect

Pat: *How do you know for sure that what you are seeing isn't just the placebo effect? After all, it's responsible for improvements in health in every single clinical drug trial. Surely LCH is likely to include some placebo in its successes.*

Me: First of all, I would never refer to it as 'just the placebo effect'. It's very powerful, extremely important and beneficial to many people. It's just that we don't know exactly how to harness it and deliver it, although we do have some ideas and some clues to help us.

Maybe there was some placebo effect in this treatment. Maybe it was all down to placebo effect. I don't know.

But I would only expect the placebo effect to bring improvements in the symptom I've been treating. Neither Clare nor I had any reason to expect her sleep to improve as a result of treatment, and yet it did.

Pat: *That could just have been a coincidence.*

Me: True, but she hadn't made any other changes at the time and she seemed to be putting it down to her treatment.

Pat: *Ok, so how could that be? How would you explain that treating her eating and her weight could lead to improvements in her sleep?*

Me: Remember that with LCH, we are digging up the roots of the weeds. It's a bit easier to think of a tree with many branches, an unwanted tree. We treated her weight and the first change was in her eating habits. If it was purely placebo, then I don't understand how or why her eating pattern changed. These habits improved, as did her sleep. We had dug up the roots of that tree, and as all three symptoms had improved, they must have all been branches off the same tree. Sometimes they're on different trees.

> **Improving the eating patterns before causing the weight to reduce is an example, for me, of LCH and the subconscious mind working together like an experienced architect and a reputable building firm. They get the foundations right, do things in the right order and at the most effective pace.**

Pat: *So is that why you have to be so careful about defining exactly what you're treating. If they were on different trees and you treated them together, then would you end up going round and round in circles?*

Me: Yes, that's right.

Pat: *I still think the sleep could have been a coincidence.*

Me: I like your healthy scepticism but there are a few other 'coincidences' in the other case studies, and you may reach a point where the weight of evidence tips in favour of there being a consistent pattern that needs to be studied in order to be explained and understood.

Clare's thoughts - the Interview

In July 2012, she spent over an hour with me, answering my questions and giving me her own personal reactions from that longer perspective.

During treatment, she had told herself to have an open mind and to just go with how she felt – and to do her homework, which involved about 20 minutes a day putting her feet up and letting the CD of my voice drone away in the background. She wasn't going to try to control her eating like she had in the past, but instead just wait and observe.

And the results – comparing before with after

She still hates to waste food, but deals with the whole situation differently now. She cooks smaller amounts, plans more and shops only for the amounts she plans to use, so there's much less to go to waste.

She mainly eats meat or fish, vegetables, salad and fruit and now can't remember the last time she wanted or ate a biscuit or bread. She consciously tries to eat more healthily, as she had many times in the past, but this time it's working and it takes no effort, no struggle, no willpower. She doesn't feel deprived in any way.

Part way through the treatment and with her habit of eating what she wanted, but without any other changes to account for it, she found that her weight was beginning to stabilise. Her weekly weigh-in was beginning to show no gains in weight and it started to reduce towards the end of her treatment sessions.

She knew that something substantial had changed. Her eating pattern had become more and more established as she got used to feeling full and satisfied on far less than she used to comfortably eat prior to treatment. And then she enjoyed the first glimpse that her weight was beginning to respond.

Quite early on, she noticed the first change in her behaviour and in how she felt. She had been to Whitby, a beautiful fishing village and tourist resort in the north east of England. It's famous for some of the freshest, locally caught fish and expertly cooked chips in the country. There are cafes and takeaways on every corner to delight the palette if you're that way inclined.

She was eating her normal sea-side day-trip treat that day, and began to feel a bit full. That alone was note-worthy. Not only did she feel full in that cafe that day, but she also knew that, if she ate another mouthful, she would then go out into the fresh sea air for a stroll along the beach, but wouldn't enjoy it that much because her stomach would feel over full of rich and heavy food. She knew that feeling very well from many similar previous day-trips.

There were several differences this time. It crossed her mind, during the meal, that she had had enough. She found herself effortlessly putting down her knife and fork. She knew, with confidence, that she would soon be happily and comfortably feasting her senses on the refreshing sea breezes, the familiar cries of the seagulls, the glint of the sunshine on the sea, and maybe even, that bracing and invigorating sting of North Sea waves on her feet and ankles as she paddled.

Me: Maybe she was seeing the first green shoots that hinted that her long bleak almost life-long winter blues of a constant battle with her eating and her weight might be moving aside to allow a comfortingly warmer and brighter spring to take hold.

Pat: *Are you letting your imagination take over? It sounds a bit over the top to me.*

Me: Remember her first contact with me - '...*Because of my weight depression is now becoming an issue*...' Others have contacted me when tears of frustration and despair have overwhelmed them.

Anyone who has never struggled in the way Clare has might wonder if I'm being overly dramatic and sensationalising a much smaller and simpler story. Any one individual choice, biscuit or not, creamy dessert or fruit, is trivial to those who don't suffer in this way.

Anyone who recognises Clare's story because it resembles their own will know that it is easy to have strong feelings in the circumstances.

Chris: *Yes, I agree. I'd be feeling those kinds of strong emotions. I also know that, because I'm overweight myself, if I go to a cafe and order any kind of treat with my tea or coffee, I sense the disapproval of anyone who isn't overweight and has noticed what I'm eating.*

Pat: *That's silly. No-one cares what a stranger is eating. People aren't criticising you or looking down on you.*

Chris: *Maybe no-one else is paying attention or judging me, but it feels like they are. I have friends who feel the same. Sometimes we go out together so it's easier to ignore those around us and we can have an occasional treat without beating ourselves up over it.*

Pat: *So if Clare felt that way too, then I suppose it was quite a relief for her.*

While she found herself reducing her portion sizes, she found herself wondering if it would last. She gained a new level of confidence in it once she had lost her first 2 or 3 lbs.

Over a longer period, the first few months after the last treatment session, that growing self-belief led her to reassess some of her eating habits consciously. She replaced sandwiches with fruit for lunch. Her regular breakfast of cereal, and buttered toast or buttered teacake or buttered crumpets was swapped for plain yoghurt and muesli.

Her main meal of meat or fish, vegetables or salad was now accompanied by a jacket potato with no butter. She's back to fish once a week, like before. That was just a phase she went through. She now skims extra fat off casseroles, cuts visible fat off bacon and other meat. She grills, doesn't fry, and uses spray-fat to reduce the amount of oil absorbed. She eats less butter and cream in general, and where appropriate, uses natural yoghurt instead.

Choosing, now, not to eat while watching TV, she enjoys her food and wants to experience those tastes and textures rather than graze absent-mindedly and miss those pleasant sensations.

She expects that she would feel sickly if she were to eat the quantity of food and the proportion of fat that she used to absorb routinely and comfortably prior to her treatment.

She has been making conscious decisions and doing what she wanted to do. She hasn't told herself she couldn't have any particular food so she hasn't been feeling deprived. Her appetite tells her when to stop.

She still enjoys her food and her social life, although some of her nearest and dearest have had to get used to a slightly different response from her. On the first post-treatment visit with her friend to their favourite fish restaurant, when the waiter arrived, Clare asked for her fish to be only lightly battered and to be served with peas, no chips. Her friend was shocked and exclaimed "But you've got to have chips!"

But no – Clare didn't have to - she didn't want to. She didn't feel deprived and enjoyed her chosen meal in the company of her friend who was tucking in to her more traditional plateful.

There is still a bottle of wine on the go at the weekend, she still eats as much as she wants, and is, to date, still losing, on average, about half a 1lb a week. Over a longer period, since she started to lose weight about 6 months ago, to date, she has lost 15.5 lbs.

She feels happier with herself. Now, she is beginning to live her life more the way she was meant to.

I believe that we're all meant to be healthy and happy, to get better at whatever we aim to learn. I do the work that I do because I believe that, in many cases, we fall off that happy, healthy path because of something that can be corrected, if we know where and how to look and what to do with it when we find it.

Clare goes swimming regularly, and enjoys that, and is beginning to dip her toes in the aqua aerobics pool. It's a bit of a challenge at the moment, but if she can feel the benefit, then maybe she'll persist and it will become easier.

Her outlook has begun to feel more positive, with an expectation that life is improving, and that trend is going to continue. Her feeling now is, 'It might take 5 years but so what?' Her target weight, the healthy body mass index, a dress size from a generation or so ago, these milestones are not around the next corner.

But neither is that disheartening yo-yo of diet and relapse, disappointment and regret.

    Pat: *Just a minute! She had 10 sessions with you. That sounds an awful lot of time and money just to lose some weight.*

Chris: *I wouldn't refer to it as 'just losing weight' because it's a huge matter for lots of us. You are very lucky not to suffer in that way, Pat. But I agree in one way. I've seen adverts where people can change their eating habits in 3 or 4 sessions. Why did it take 10 sessions? Why had she only lost a few pounds in all that time?*

    Me: Most people, living with this aspect of their lives, simply want to lose weight. But if you scratch the surface a bit, you often find that it's affecting them in many more ways. Food is on their mind from the moment they wake up. That sense of failure, that feeling of being judged, they feel their own and everyone else's disappointment in themselves.

If there's tempting food in the house, whether it's chocolate or crisps or biscuits, whether it's fairly ordinary treats or snacks for the children or a special present for Grandma, there's an almighty battle raging in the person's head which never stops until that food is gone.

If the food is gone because they gave in and ate it, then as well as having to go out and replace the food without anyone noticing, there's that guilt and remorse and regret that is so painful

and needs the comfort and pain relief of yet
more of that tempting food.

In a restaurant, served a plate of food far bigger
than is needed, that plate of food seems to be in
control. Just like the chocolate and biscuits that
call out from the cupboard and the ice-cream
that yells from the freezer, there's no rest from
that state of powerlessness. What sort of life is
it when something inanimate and seemingly
benign has such an iron grip on our behaviour
and our thoughts and our feelings?

Look at what has changed for Clare. Without
any effort, habits have changed. Who would
have thought that, after clearing her plate every
mealtime for over 50 years, that habit would
disappear mysteriously in fewer than 50 days?

Remember what you said before I started this
account of Clare's treatment. Pat, you said
*"That would certainly fit a 'magic wand' kind
of fairy story for me. It sounds too farfetched.
I don't believe that ever really happens. Decades
of habits don't just reverse themselves in a few
weeks and months"*. And Chris, you said,
*"I agree and I'm not interested in fiction. Tell us
what really happened."*

Pat: *I'd forgotten that. Yes you're right.*

Chris: *Hmmm...*

Me: People have come to me for treatment having
completed one of those '3 or 4 session' therapies
because they need 'a top up'. They go back,

68

about once a year, because the effort they had to make to lose the weight was getting harder and harder. They never actually reached that state where they felt full and naturally stopped eating. It was just that it didn't require quite so much effort.

Pat: *Do you mean that people come to you expecting another top up and then learn that LCH is completely different from the other therapies they have tried?*

Me: Yes, that has happened. Some have come to me because their previous therapist was unavailable or they decided to try someone else for some reason.

Even if losing weight requires just a small amount of effort, it will eventually wear us down. If it happens automatically, then it's totally effort-free. It isn't even being noticed by us.

Thinking about your magic wand answers when we first started discussing Clare's treatment, the changes I described were beyond your imagination. You saw it as fiction. And yet you are still surprised at how many sessions were needed.

Chris: *I wouldn't have predicted it. And yes, such an experience is well worth the number of sessions it took to achieve it.*

Pat: *You've helped me to see it more clearly and I agree it's more than 'just losing weight'.*

Me: I can remember thinking, during the initial consultation, how good it would feel when she learnt that it hadn't been a life sentence after all.

She can comfortably look in the mirror now, and is getting rid of older clothes that are too big for her now. Those that still have some life in them, she is taking the time to get out the needle and cotton and take them in at the seams.

Once we reached the stage where it seemed clear that no further treatment was needed, we agreed to check in once a month for an update. If she began to struggle at any point with the decisions, the choices about healthy food or the ease with which she stopped eating once full, if she stopped feeling full after a reasonably sized meal, then we would need to check for any previously hidden stray roots.

I don't believe that I can ever be 100% certain that every last trace has gone. I do believe that any remaining issues can be as easily and quickly resolved as the main ones were.

Chris: *That sounds awfully expensive! That's a lot of treatment and a lot of money!*

Pat: *Yes, and what were you treating?*

Me: The check-in was in the form of a quick phone call or email, which would have only taken a few minutes. There was no further treatment and no further charge after session 10.

Pat: *And do you do that with everyone, that ongoing 'checking in' process?*

Me: No, it's quite rare for me to do that, but with certain conditions, like weight loss, where someone has a need to lose quite a lot of weight and a healthy rate of weight loss is quite slow, then treatment is likely to be completed quite a few months before that desired healthy weight is reached.

Also, people tell me of diets they've been on where they've lost weight, as much as they wanted or needed to, and then, slowly, steadily, the weight creeps back on. In order to show people how different the experience with LCH can be, a much longer history is needed.

Clare agreed to let me tell her story and the pre-publication update shows the best information yet available on just how valuable was the time and money spent on those 10 sessions.

Her cholesterol, in April 2011, was 8.2. In April 2012, it had gone down to 5.1, presumably because of the changes in her diet. That's yet another benefit for her health and wellbeing and peace of mind. Fantastic!

Now in her mid 60's with a history of many years of more weight, extra body fat than would be ideal for her physical health, it's not surprising that she had got quite used to some ongoing, grumbling aches and pains. Those are also reducing. Oh joy!

Her knee still hurts but not quite as much, and I'm confident that this slow and steady reduction in her weight should eventually help that to heal, at least to some degree.

She should be spared some of the negative side-effects of rapid weight loss. Even for someone in their teens or twenties, the body struggles to adjust if the weight falls too quickly, but the effect can be much more severe as we get older.

With a weight loss of 1lb or 2lb a week combined with exercise such as walking or swimming, she is likely to enjoy only positive and healthy effects.

Pat and Chris disagree on something

Pat: *I'm not sure it's a good thing to tell people they might need to come back. If a therapist said that to me, it would make me think they'd got no confidence that I could or would respond well to treatment. I'd assume their therapy and their ability to deliver it were a bit on the weak side. It also sounds like a money-making scheme.*

Chris: *I disagree. It sounds reassuring to me. If I went to the doctor for some treatment and they said they wanted to see me again in 6 months' time to monitor progress, I'd think they were being thorough and taking care of me. We all respond differently to whatever kind of treatment or therapy we have, and I feel unsettled if someone seems to be confidently predicting what I don't think they can possibly know – how I am going to progress. I'd also feel nervous about contacting that same therapist because*

I wouldn't know how they would respond. I'd worry they might take it badly in some way, like if someone asks for a second opinion and the doctor feels their expertise is being questioned.

Me: You've highlighted a subject I've heard discussed before, and on the whole, although it's only a small sample, most of the therapists – LCH and non-LCH hypnotherapists – seemed to agree with you, Pat. On the other hand, people I have treated and some other people I have discussed it with seem to be more in agreement with Chris's view.

I also agree with Chris, on balance. I can see value in both viewpoints but, on the whole, see it as better for most people in most circumstances to offer what I intend as reassurance. I would consider each client individually in this decision, and if I thought it better for any one client, then I would adjust my explanations accordingly.

I will continue to listen to people's opinions for and against and will change my default plan if, on balance, I ever decide that that's what's best for my clients.

Clare's overview of her treatment

She didn't think any symptom–focussed treatment or therapy would have worked because she believes she would have continued to have that exhausting struggle, that battle of wills that the subconscious always wins in the long run. She expects that she would also have continued to suffer that deprived feeling, which had always worn down her resolve in the past.

She hung on in there for quite a few weeks before she saw any signs of improvement in her weight. She had been assisted in her decision to keep going by the experiences she had with her improved eating patterns.

She had gained a little weight in November 2011 but her eating patterns had continued to improve. She had continued to monitor the situation, wondering whether to keep on with the treatment. Having gone this far and having spent this money, she would certainly give it more time. After all, something could be just around the corner. In fact, she felt sure it would be, and either way, she felt like she had nothing else to try.

As another resource to help the process along, I had lent her a copy of my first book 'What if it really is...?'. She had read it with interest and the ideas she found there made a lot of sense to her. If there had been some real life stories included, that would probably have helped her even more.

That first experience of fish and chips at Whitby had really surprised her. Knowing that she would have felt disappointed in herself, and also a bit sickly, and finding it easy to leave food on her plate were all experiences that were refreshingly unfamiliar and most welcome.

New habits are becoming more and more ingrained. She still doesn't waste food, but has found a better place to store it until it's needed. She puts the extra in the fridge now for that night's supper or for lunch the next day, rather than carrying it around with her on her hips, her waistline and her thighs.

She told me that, if she had read 'What if' before she had come to see me, she doesn't think she would have been quite so sceptical. She hung on in there with her treatment as an act of faith and with no other avenue available to her, but if she had known more about it, she believes she would have found the decision to carry on much easier.

Knowing how habits of many decades can change in a matter of a few weeks or months can help people decide whether to consider LCH as a promising option. She can imagine that many people will identify with her 'before' experiences, and if reading her chapters will help them see that her 'after' experiences are possible for them too, then she is more than happy for me to tell her story.

Update in June 2013

I contacted Clare for an interim update and leant that she is still getting on fine, still losing weight slowly and feels that that's ok. It takes no effort and she hardly ever even thinks about it now. At first it was always in her thoughts.

She wondered if there was any likelihood of a relapse, of old habits and concerns returning and was reassured to hear that I believe it's unlikely but that a few more sessions would be likely to fix it easily if there were any kind of 'wobble'.

Her treatment with me still comes to mind from time to time, though, when she finds herself throwing clothes away that are too big for her now, and scraping left-over food into the bin. She has taken in 2 pairs of trousers recently because they were too big but too new to throw away.

I don't think I could bear to force myself to finish a meal if it was too much, now.

Best money I ever spent!

And the latest update, from February 2014, is a total loss of 2stone 4lbs from her pre-treatment weight.

Me: Pat and Chris, what are the main messages for you from this case?

Chris: *It seems like Pat and I, and even Clare herself, have been taken by surprise. A habit of 50 years or more just changing almost overnight, without any effort, isn't something many people would expect to happen. The kind of habits she had take time to create and then normally just seem to get more and more embedded and sticky and resistant to all attempts to shift them.*

Pat: *Yes, but that's when we try to work on our own, just using the willpower of the conscious mind. When we work together with the subconscious mind, maybe we can start to expect a more powerful result.*

CHAPTER 5

The freedom to be gained is worth far more than the cost of the sessions

Pat, Chris and I discuss and agree what to focus on next

Chris: *Now tell us about the person who wanted to give up smoking. I've tried a few times to give up and haven't succeeded yet. You might have another client if you can convince me that you can help me to stop.*

Pat: *Yes, that's one I'm quite puzzled about because I've seen loads of adverts claiming to make you a non-smoker in a single session, and that doesn't sound like something you would do. So I really want to know what you did and how it went. Was there an underlying cause?*

Me: I've seen those adverts too. They tend to include some form of guarantee. Some offer free further treatment in the unlikely event that that single session isn't completely successful.

Pat: *It doesn't sound like something the LCH College would teach because, from what you've told us,*

you can't possibly find and resolve an underlying
cause in one session using LCH techniques.

Me: There is an anti-smoking technique taught on
the Practical Course and it is a single-session
treatment using direct instructions and
suggestions.

Pat: *Why is that? It doesn't seem to fit with LCH.*

Me: It doesn't seem to fit with me either. I don't
offer that kind of treatment even though I've
had the training, and even though, as far as
I know, many LCH therapists offer it when
appropriate.

Pat: *What do you mean by 'when appropriate'?*

Me: I can't really answer for those therapists who
offer it, but as far as I understand it, they look
for signs of a simple smoking habit that started
due to peer pressure as a teenager. Anything
other than that, like addictions to any other
substances or behaviours like heavy drinking
of alcohol or problem gambling, or signs of
severe anxiety, would probably lead to LCH
treatment being offered instead. If the smoker
is using their habit to keep themselves calm,
to help themselves cope with normal day-to-
day life, that would probably mean that the
therapist would decide that the single-session
treatment was inappropriate.

Pat: *Why is cigarette smoking seen as something*
different from other forms of addiction?

Me: Again, I can't really answer, because the reasoning that I heard on the course didn't convince me.

Pat: *So you just don't offer that service?*

Me: That's correct.

Pat: *Aren't you worried that that is letting your clients down?*

Me: No. I don't lose any sleep over it. There are plenty of people offering that kind of treatment, so if anyone wants that service, they will easily be able to find another therapist who is willing and able to deliver it for them. There are far fewer LCH therapists, so I believe my time is better spent on specialising in that work.

Pat: *So what do you do if someone comes to you to stop smoking? What do you say to them?*

Me: I don't see many, probably because most therapists who offer it will highlight that offer in their advertising. Among those people who want to give up smoking, most of them will search specifically for a specialist in that area. Since I started in 2006, I've only had a few people come to me to stop smoking.

Pat: *So did you do your normal treatment?*

Me: Yes, and I'm so glad I did. But I did find myself thinking and re-considering many times before I got to that point. The first time I found myself facing someone who wanted my help to give up smoking, I can remember wondering what sort of response I would get and trusting that my instincts were guiding me in the best direction for my client.

Pat: *How many sessions did that person have altogether?*

Me: 14

Pat: *14 sessions to stop smoking! You won't get people queuing up to see you on that kind of performance, will you?*

Me: No, but there was a bit more to it than that.

Pat: *Well I hope there was, because that's an awful lot of time and money for something that seems quite straight-forward.*

Me: What do you think, Chris? As a smoker yourself, do you agree with Pat?

Chris: *Hmmm... If it works completely, then the cost of those sessions will be paid for in a matter of months if the smoker was on 20 a day. If the habit goes and the cravings go as well, then the peace of mind and freedom from that nagging voice, that morning cough, that smell that surrounds you, the health risks, the signal it sends to the children.... it's worth far more than the cost of 14 sessions.*

Pat: *Ok. I guess I need to think a bit more about the full effects of symptoms I don't suffer from if I'm going to eventually become a therapist. I'll bear that in mind as you take us through the treatment.*

It seems like you disagree quite a lot with your LCH colleagues as well as with other kinds of hypnotherapists. Shouldn't you be trying to work out who is right? Do people get annoyed when you're always putting forward a different point of view?

Me: No. My colleagues in LCH and my hypnotherapy colleagues of all different philosophies seem to agree, in general, that debate and discussion is healthy. We are more likely to progress that way. By keeping our minds and our problem-solving skills as sharp and honed as possible, we're going to be even better at providing a reliable and efficient service to our clients.

Pat: *It sounds like I'm going to need to learn to think more for myself and be less reliant on what experts tell me.*

Chris: *Does it make a difference to how you treat someone if they're addicted to more than one thing, like smoking and drinking or binge-eating or gambling?*

Me: Well, what do you think? Should I treat them all at once or one at a time?

Pat: *I think that, if you treat them one at a time, that when the first one you treat starts to improve, the other addiction will probably increase to fill the space left by the decreasing one.*

Chris: *Yes, I can imagine that happening too.*

Pat: *So if that's what happens, then maybe, treating them all at once would be better.*

Me: So keep that thought in mind as I take you through it, session by session.

Let me introduce...

We need to rewind a bit first. The story starts in the spring of 2009, a few months before I first met Cathy. I went to a networking meeting and, when it came to my turn, I did my one-minute introduction, something I understand the networking community call an 'elevator pitch'. I'd be most impressed if someone could do justice to the story of LCH in one minute.

Cathy's husband was at the meeting, and he probably wasn't able to take much relevant information home with him that day. He just picked up my name and my job and, at the end of the session, asked me for a business card. That's it. He didn't ask me any questions, didn't volunteer any information except to say that his wife wanted to give up smoking.

Cathy saw that business card in the pile of cards and leaflets that her husband cleared out of his pockets that night. She picked up the card and emailed me to make an appointment. Out of all the cards, leaflets, magazine articles, local advertising magazine listings and web search results she will have had at her disposal at the time, something made her choose to get in touch with me.

When I interviewed her for this chapter, I was even more surprised to find that her expectations about what treatment would involve were very different from how I deliver treatment. She hadn't seen my leaflet or my website. She had simply sent an email to the address on the card. She had expected a single session of direct suggestions along the lines of "you will never smoke another cigarette" and "you will never feel the urge to light up ever again".

In spite of the fact that Cathy doesn't have faith in quick fixes, and in spite of the fact that she had expected that that would be what I would provide, she still came along to see me. I don't know where she might have got a clue, but maybe some instinct drove her to ring my number. She was very pleased and relieved to hear that my way of working was so much more in line with what she wanted and could believe in.

CHAPTER 6

The subconscious is always working in that conscientious, ethical and loving way

Session 1

The consultation

I got a few basic details from Cathy. She was in her 50's, married, with 3 grown up children. She wanted to give up smoking. She was about to become a grandmother and didn't want to expose her grandchildren to the smell of stale smoke. It's a simple enough request and a common one for most hypnotherapists to receive.

Her smoking history

She started at 14 years old and continued until she was 23. Many people find it relatively easy to give up with the incentive of the improved health of their new family. She didn't completely stop but she didn't smoke much. She never smoked around her babies and young children. She just had the occasional one or two on those rare and precious nights out as a young mum off duty and letting her hair down.

Most of the time when she was smoking very little, she was much fitter and healthier. She enjoyed exercising, walking and running. She had an ectopic pregnancy in her 30's and had to stop exercising while she recovered from that. Puzzlingly, although she had previously enjoyed feeling active, had liked to stretch her legs and take in the fresh air and the sunshine, once she had fully recovered from the ectopic pregnancy, she found she couldn't summon up the enthusiasm and motivation to start exercising again.

At 42, she started smoking again. Things had got on top of her and the cigarettes seemed to help her cope with increasing levels of stress.

How it was affecting her

She smoked as a reward for a job well done, as a treat when she'd been working hard, as a crutch when she needed something to lean on, when she was looking for relief, for comfort. It was the first thing she thought about on waking and the last thing she had to do at night.

She had a responsible and stressful job and smoked to help herself get there in the morning, smoking 2 or 3 before work, 2 or 3 during breaks and the rest to help her unwind when she got home and last thing at night before going to bed.

She could go for hours without a cigarette, especially when around non-smokers, but then would light up, sometimes without really knowing why.

Why she wanted to give up

She wished she had never started smoking, especially as being a smoker seemed to sap her self-confidence. She is strong-willed in most aspects of life but hadn't managed to beat this particular habit.

She hated smelling of stale cigarette smoke.

The cost was another nudge. She resented and begrudged the relentless and significant drain on her finances as a result of her habit.

She was aware how unhealthy and antisocial it's now seen to be and was tired of having to go out and buy more if she ever allowed herself to run out before the end of the day.

She especially didn't want to give that example to her grandchildren, didn't want them to ever see her smoking.

What she had tried so far

Like most reluctant smokers, she had tried willpower and nicotine patches. Both had provided some good results but they never lasted long. As a testament to her strength of will and determination, she has managed to stop for a few months, but then lost the momentum, gave up on that constant battle against those urges and that little voice.... "Go on, you can have one now. It's been 3 days since your last one so you're clearly not addicted. You can just smoke when you want to. And why shouldn't you have something you enjoy?"

She used the nicotine patches, and had no real problems with them, except that they didn't stop her from smoking. She just ended up taking in even more nicotine.

How I could help

I explained to Cathy that I could work with her subconscious, the part controlling and maintaining her smoking habit. I could help that part of her mind to reach a solution that is better for her as a whole, physically, mentally and emotionally, consciously and subconsciously.

I didn't make a note of exactly what I said, how I explained, because my treatment notes are focussed totally on what is relevant for treatment. When writing in more detail, for a wider audience, there are some pieces of information that it would be useful to have a record of, but at the time of treating Cathy, and all the rest of the case study subjects, I had no idea that their stories would form the core of my second book.

I probably painted a picture of the subconscious as behaving like that nurturing, caring parent taking their child to the doctor's for an injection. The parent knows that it will hurt and the child will be scared, but believes that, in the long run, it's for the best. They take guidance from the best medical advice available at the time. They believe in the benefits of an immunisation against a childhood disease that could otherwise cause severe, long-term or even permanent damage. The parent is guided by the best science around and reassures the child and encourages them to be brave.

Although many people have differing views about the safety and effectiveness of immunisation for the individual, my use of it as an analogy here is based on an assumption that, in general, parents follow NHS advice while their children are too young to decide for themselves.

Some of those immunisation programmes have been halted over the generations because of evidence emerging of severe side-effects being suffered in some cases. The Polio Programme and the MMR combined vaccine are memorable examples of concern over observed correlations with severe worrying symptoms and illnesses. More research was needed to learn whether the correlation was also a causation and people watched and waited for a while until clearer evidence emerged. Where we learnt there was no causation, we were advised to resume the programme and where there was causation, better and safer medication was developed and then the programme was resumed.

Cathy remembered me explaining that the subconscious makes sure we turn over in bed when we're asleep, and does that most of the time without waking us. That

measure prevents pressure sores from developing.
We would need nursing care to do that turning for
us if we were so deeply unconscious that it wasn't
happening automatically. She also remembers we mulled
over that experience of driving on a long and familiar
journey when we sometimes arrive without actually
realising how we got there. We're driving on autopilot,
conscious mind off duty, subconscious at the wheel
and keeping us safe. Both of those examples fit with a
nurturing parent image.

How this could explain a habit like smoking, with all
its known health risks, being part of what a nurturing
subconscious might create - one of my colleagues
summed it up well. Faced with a crisis, the subconscious
needs to prioritise, so although, in this case, smoking is
generally seen as significantly harmful to our health, the
subconscious must believe there's an even greater risk or
an even stronger need.

I believe the subconscious is always working in that
conscientious, ethical and loving way. For some
reason, at that time, Cathy's subconscious believed
she needed that smoking habit. That reason might be
based on some long-forgotten information which might
now be out of date, or might have been misunderstood
at the time.

It's important to gain the confidence of the subconscious
mind that the treatment always remains under its
control and that I'm not aiming to take over and impose
any changes from outside. If that confidence leads to
collaboration, leads to the subconscious mind working

with me, I can help guide the process of investigation and re-examination of that information.

That re-examination could result in some re-processing, re-calibrating, re-interpretation, and the final effects of all of that will be that, if the habit is no longer needed, the subconscious will take it away. In general, once it becomes clear that the habit isn't in the client's best interest, the subconscious disposes of it readily, just as Clare's did with her plate-clearing habit. It doesn't need any persuasion from me.

The decision to go ahead

Cathy was happy that what I said made sense to her and we agreed to make a start there and then.

Her previous experience of hypnotherapy

She hadn't had any previous experience of hypnosis or hypnotherapy and was curious as to how it would feel. She had heard my explanations, describing it as very similar to the kind of relaxation you might achieve when chilling out listening to music or lying in bed on a Sunday morning, enjoying the comfort and happy not to have to get up just yet. She just needed to experience that for herself.

The first experience of hypnosis

She put her feet up with a mix of expectations and experienced a pleasant light and subtle relaxation.

Looking back on it, she told me of her surprise at how much she was able to hear and how much she felt in control. She felt like she could just open her eyes and sit up at any time, which she hadn't expected, and didn't actually do. She had felt safe knowing that she retained that control throughout. She knew she was able to end the session at any point, but she didn't want to and really couldn't be bothered to test it out.

Homework - CD Practice

I explained about her homework, what she needed to do and why. She needed to take home a CD after each session and play it once a day, or nearly every day. She would get to put her feet up and be off-duty for about 20 minutes a day relaxing to the sound of my voice.

Some of the messages in the CD's I use are designed to reassure the conscious mind, to remind them of explanations given during the consultation. They supply information relevant to the subconscious mind too. The subconscious has gone to a lot of trouble to create a habit for the client's own good and needs to be reassured that treatment is in her best interest.

The client needs to learn a new way of responding during treatment sessions. We tend to listen when someone speaks to us. We tend to think about what they are saying to us before we respond. I need to help my clients learn to steadily reduce the conscious mind's control of that conversation by beginning to allow a kind of 'off-duty' state to develop.

It takes a while for that new way of responding to become established, which is great because I need a degree of conscious involvement in sessions 2 and 3, the early stages of treatment. I need the conscious mind to hand over the microphone to the subconscious mind, and I need the subconscious mind to be willing and able to step forward and communicate with me.

This is how a colleague explains it – clearly and to the point.

There is a process that takes place between the first and third sessions. This process helps the patient to gently move from initially experiencing hypnosis (relaxation) in Session One to eventually providing me the subconscious information I need. Achieving this in just one session would be difficult, if not impossible, so there is a very tightly constructed series of steps that helps the patient to gradually become more and more adept at doing so. In session 2 I begin to introduce the patient to answering some simple questions. Some of these answers are highly likely to be conscious at first, but after a little practice and some additional easy to follow instructions, subconscious answers begin to occur, and this paves the way for all future sessions. By the third session the patient is usually well on his way to providing subconscious answers.

The CD practice is designed to progressively guide and facilitate that development. I need my clients to be prepared to play their part. I can't do this on my own. We need to work together.

Cathy went home with her CD and instructions of how to practise.

Session 2 – one week later

How the CD practice had gone

She had practised most days and her attention had begun to wander quite naturally. I didn't need to explain any more except to reassure her that all was going well from that point of view.

Any more information

The discussion in session 1 often causes clients to find that other aspects of their symptom come to mind and we go through those at the start of session 2. Also, the way things are explained in the consultation can lead to a client wondering if LCH could be beneficial for something else that is bothering them. We had both of these with Cathy.

She had started smoking as a young teenager, with 5 of her friends, but none of the rest had gone on to smoke regularly, so she might have experienced peer-pressure to try it out, but was under no pressure to continue. She had and the other 5 hadn't, so something must have caused her to respond differently from the rest.

Cathy has had backache for more than 20 years. It has been diagnosed as sciatica. There is a sharp spasm from time to time, and a dull ache almost always there in the background. She's had medical tests but no treatment that has resolved it and she didn't know of any reason for it other than general wear and tear. I made a note of that and suggested that that might be something we could usefully investigate once the smoking was resolved.

Memories recalled

During the hypnosis, a memory came back from her early childhood, but it wasn't one that had any logical connection to smoking, so that told me that she hadn't consciously searched her memories for something relevant. She had found herself imagining a scene without knowing why. She hadn't chosen it, so her subconscious must have. That means to me that her subconscious was already beginning to work with me, to play its part, to give me information.

Any further CD guidance

I gave her another CD and the same instructions on how to practise, and Cathy went home.

Session 3 –10 days later

CD progress

The CD practice was going well. Cathy was finding herself relaxed and mentally drifting off into other thoughts and daydreams. She didn't need any extra advice or help. So far, things seemed to be coming naturally to her.

The treatment

We worked on the first few clues about her smoking habit, about why it had become ingrained. We work quite a lot with closed questioning, questions just requiring a Yes/No answer to make it as easy as possible for the answers to be instinctive.

Imagine a teenager watching their favourite TV programme or engrossed in emails, social media or computer games. Mum wants to know if he's done his homework and if he wants egg and chips for tea. Over the years, he and his subconscious mind have developed between them the answers that will most quickly get Mum to go away and leave him in peace and that will ensure he gets to regularly eat his most favourite food. With hardly a split second gap in his focus on the screen, all the most appropriate Yes's and No's just seem to come out of his mouth.

Cathy was too relaxed to fully monitor the questions, to be bothered to keep track of them, and yet somehow she just instinctively knew what the answer was. She didn't have any conscious knowledge or logic or reasoning guiding her, so I believe that means the subconscious 'knew'. Everything was going well.

The next CD

She didn't need any further information to be supplied by the CD to her conscious or her subconscious mind. She just needed to keep on practising, relaxing to the sound of my voice. An automatic response was beginning to develop more and more strongly, just as it was meant to, so that as soon as I started to count, she started to relax and her attention started to wander off.

Session 4 – 3 weeks later

A couple of days before session 4 was arranged for, she rang to cancel due to illness. She assured me she would rebook when she had recovered. I knew from experience with other clients that there was a possibility that she wouldn't but had to just wait and see. I hoped she would return so that I could help her improve her chances of a long and healthy life by assisting her in her wish to quit smoking.

It generally takes more than 4 sessions

I've found, over the years, that some clients attend between 1 and 4 sessions and then cancel because of some change of plan, some work or family rearrangement of appointments, some problem with the car or a pet, and then they don't rebook. I don't know why that is, and I assume that there are several different reasons, but I have a few theories. I hope that most have simply found that their symptom has already reduced to a point where they have forgotten all about it and all about the treatment they were receiving as they get on with their busy lives.

But I don't expect that that's true for all of them. Most people who come to me for treatment have never heard of LCH. They've heard good reports about the effectiveness and ease with which hypnotherapy can eliminate unwanted habits and phobias. There are many different types of hypnotherapy, but I only have a professional knowledge and expertise in LCH itself.

As far as I understand it, some work directly on the symptom, believing the cause to be long gone and irrelevant, forgotten and best left undisturbed like that sleeping dog. Some, like LCH, believe that the cause needs to be resolved and have combined their hypnotherapy practice with some aspects of a more psychotherapeutic approach. Pure psychotherapy itself often goes on once or twice a week for many months and sometimes many years.

Those who work directly on the symptom seem to be able to predict very accurately how many sessions will be needed. Many people probably gain an impression that hypnotherapy is successful in somewhere between one and four sessions depending on the symptom being treated.

LCH needs a certain kind of counter-intuitive response that is quite different from how the conscious and subconscious parts of the mind normally interact with the outside world. The underlying cause, the hidden treasure, the key to unlock the door that leads out into symptom-free sunshine could be in an obvious place but could equally be hidden deep in a cupboard in the far corner of the cellar. For these and other reasons, three sessions are required to get all the foundations in place which facilitate gaining subconscious information.

Some of my colleagues include in their literature a guideline of 6 to 8 sessions. I don't do that because it feels like it holds a heavy weight of expectation on both me and my client to fit into that pattern, and an implied low standard or even failure if it takes more than 8 sessions.

But equally, I need my clients to know what to expect as much as I'm able to, so after the first few years in practice, I've been able to explain that a pattern seems to be emerging. At any time after session 1, the client may feel a sense of relief that a treatment they have some understanding of and a degree of confidence in, has actually started. That sense of relief on its own can cause symptoms to temporarily and partially improve. Even the CD practice, which gives a daily opportunity for 20 minutes off-duty, which many people wouldn't normally allow themselves to enjoy, can add to that early feeling of partial relief.

Somewhere around session 4 or 5 or 6, sessions usually taken on a weekly basis, there is the first breakthrough that causes a positive shift, a reduction in the symptom. From then on, I usually recommend monthly appointments until the symptom has gone completely or has shown signs of a steady improvement that the client feels confident of.

I recommend moving to monthly appointments then because it feels more efficient and effective to allow the subconscious time to do some tidying up and re-cataloguing so that it's easier to spot any remaining stray roots at the next session. I often find, during that time, that there was more than one cause, more than one set of roots that needed digging up.

Eventually, after a small number of monthly sessions, a complete search for remaining errors draws a complete blank. My client's conscious and subconscious mind both agree that all is sorted.

At that point, I advise that no further treatment is necessary, but not to be concerned if the improvement plateaus before the symptom is completely gone, or if there is a u-turn at some point.

I believe that, when a misunderstanding is found, the subconscious searches the attic, the cellar, the garage, the shed and all those cupboards and drawers in our mental and emotional house. Anything related to that misunderstanding is re-examined and where appropriate, is recycled, re-housed, goes into the compost bin or the charity bag. I also believe that that process carries on in the background long after treatment is concluded. If that's the case, then something could turn up at any time and need another look. When we sort through a pile of old, long-forgotten stuff, we can often find something that isn't necessarily out-of-date. It might actually still be needed.

The subconscious might find something like that and it might be relevant to the need for that original symptom. The subconscious might decide that it was still needed after all, and simply bring it back in again.

If that were to happen, the client might decide that LCH, like many of the other measures and remedies tried before, had only been a temporary fix. I wouldn't want to leave my clients with that possibility so I explain that if they had that kind of experience, then it's highly likely that there is another piece of information or two to re-examine, and they simply need to get in touch and come back for a few more sessions to help get it resolved.

Cathy came back

She recovered from her illness, rebooked and we resumed where we left off.

She described how, recently, she had felt as if she was asleep during CD practice, but that she had always found herself awake and alert at some point during the countdown at the end of the recording. If she had been asleep, then her subconscious had been diligent and doing its job of waking her at the appropriate time.

Sometimes, people need to put a bit of effort into playing their part in treatment. For others, it seems to just come naturally. Cathy was one of those lucky ones who find it fairly easy at first, and then notice it get even easier with each session. She was quite bemused by the way she just instinctively knew the answers to the questions without knowing why she knew. She thought it bizarre but was happy to go along with it.

Her subconscious worked with me and together we found a possibly misunderstood incident during that session's questioning and were able to agree on a more balanced and mature interpretation. Cathy was happily day-dreaming. Her subconscious mind and I were productively problem-solving, following clues, putting evidence under the microscope and agreeing on amendments and corrections to what it all might actually mean.

Symptom changes

Puzzlingly, Cathy hadn't had any urges to smoke for a few weeks. She was still using nicotine patches but didn't attribute this development to those as they hadn't worked for her before. She had known that something was different because she had been to a party, had had a few drinks but strangely hadn't felt any temptation to smoke. That was most unusual. Even with her strong will, a drink or two was usually enough to reach the 'what the heck' stage, but not that time.

I was puzzled as the improvement seemed have started before we found what seemed to be relevant information, but maybe her subconscious mind had gone on ahead and done some foraging of its own. Maybe it had just decided that the jury was out, that there was no need for Cathy to be suffering while those jurors considered their verdict. Time would tell. We left a couple of weeks between sessions this time to allow for some of that processing that follows a reassessment. The knock on effects of the original interpretation would need to be replaced by the logical follow-on effects of the recent re-evaluation.

Session 5 – 2 weeks later

Cathy arrived with yet more puzzling news. She had found herself drinking less since the previous session. I wondered if that was what she wanted because she hadn't previously mentioned alcohol as being of any concern to her at all. She had always enjoyed a few drinks but had been drinking quite a lot, quite frequently, and it had occasionally been a bit worrying if she stopped to think about it. She had, from time to time, wondered if she had some kind of drink problem but hadn't come to a decision.

As she suddenly found herself enjoying mornings without the hangover that she had become accustomed to, she realised just how much it had been affecting her, draining her energy. It had caused her to waste so many hours of her precious weekends because she had habitually felt too delicate to enjoy doing anything more than recovering from the effects of the night before.

Another development helped confirm that we were working deep down at the roots where she was likely to gain significant and long-lasting benefit. Cathy had spent many years feeling like she had to apologise for everything, that anything that went wrong must be her fault. She now felt stronger and happier, with a clearer sense that, on the whole, it wasn't her fault.

But what she came to me for – the smoking?

Since the last session she had felt the urge to test out her new freedom from cravings to smoke. I was so pleased to hear that she hadn't enjoyed the experience and that it hadn't set her off again just yet. I've heard other therapists report that a single cigarette can undo the effects of the single-session treatment but I hadn't heard if the same happened with LCH treatment for smoking.

Cathy was happy to report that no harm had been done and that, on the contrary, it had given her the confidence that she had been wanting. She now knew, as a result of that test, that it wasn't a quick fix that might break again later. She strongly believed that the addiction was gone.

But it's not just up to her. The subconscious mind is most in charge of habits and addictions and cravings and urges. I needed to ask some questions and I needed pure subconscious information. She was finding it easier and easier to respond instinctively, to not care about the questions, to not give them a thought but just supply the automatic Yes or No each time. The subconscious information confirmed her opinion that the addiction had been removed. I checked as meticulously as I could for any remaining stray roots. There didn't seem to be any. The habit wasn't needed any more.

But neither of us wanted to leave it there. It didn't feel like there had been enough time to be sure. We agreed to book another session in about a month's time. I felt that there might be more ways she could benefit and she wanted to gain more confidence that this wasn't a temporary phenomenon.

Session 6 – 4 weeks later

She hadn't smoked or used any nicotine patches since the previous session. There were no cravings or urges to smoke, so she hadn't needed to make any effort. She seemed to have put her smoking days behind her.

That previous guilt was also still gone. She was beginning to find herself able to say no to other people's requests for her help when she wanted or needed to. She no longer felt obliged to put others first as if she owed it to them. She was finding a more balanced way of dealing with her own needs and rights in the face of the wants and needs of others.

We went on to consider other symptoms including the backache she had mentioned in an earlier session.

She had also noticed some weight gain since she had stopped smoking. As well as the continued reduction in her underlying sense of guilt, she still wasn't drinking alcohol, neither of which had been addressed at any time in her treatment, so the weight gain was puzzling.

But Cathy didn't seem concerned about the weight gain at all. She wanted to work on the backache, which we did. The information pointed to it having the same underlying cause as the smoking and it looked like that would also begin to improve, but there might be more to it.

More recently, she learned that she has an under-active thyroid and believes this could have been developing for quite a while, and might have led to the mysterious weight gain.

Session 7 – 3 weeks later

She had some slight reduction in the spasms and the dull ache and we continued the investigation, but the answers weren't quite so forthcoming that session. It seemed like her subconscious was busy with all we'd done in previous sessions and wasn't ready yet for any further work.

But there was yet another surprise in store. Cathy had suffered from excessive underarm sweating that wasn't due to physical exertion. It was more like a blushing response. That embarrassing damp patch under the arm had often let her down in work and social situations in the past. She had noticed, over the previous few weeks, that that had also gone away.

Maybe the puzzling weight gain was part of the process of fixing the sweating. If I'm going to have a new kitchen fitted, then there's going to be a lot of mess and noise and upheaval, especially if there is some extra pipe-work and drainage to sort out before the new units can be built. In the work that I've done with the subconscious up to now, when I've finally gained all the relevant information, it eventually always makes perfect sense. It inevitably confirms the theory that that part of the mind was always doing, and will always do, its best for us.

Session 8 – 3 weeks later

Nothing else emerged that session except for repeated confirmation that all was going well and that the backache would go.

Session 9 – 6 weeks later

Cathy still hadn't wanted or smoked a single cigarette since that test a few months previously.

She was still drinking little if any alcohol and seeing that as a bonus. It was like how she had felt at 11 years old when it would never have crossed her mind that she wanted or needed a drink or a smoke.

The backache was reducing, with no spasms at all for a few months and the dull ache had changed more to a feeling of stiffness.

The guilt was becoming a distant memory. She was pleased to find that she still cared, that she hadn't become unfeeling, but how refreshing to be able to empathise with other people without feeling the weight of guilt for their pain and without a responsibility to take it away for them. She could listen and be supportive but only help them if it was right for her as well as for them.

With such noticeable reduction in the backache and 3 sessions of searching which hadn't shown any signs of any other underlying causes, we agreed to leave that to continue improving and work instead on her weight.

The weight gain seemed to be based on the same information as the smoking, the alcohol and the excessive sweating, so I wasn't able to fully make sense of why it had emerged as the smoking stopped. Any number of hypotheses come to mind, like my kitchen scenario.

Or maybe the subconscious had responded to the first reassessment by transferring to another path, without noticing at the time, that it was still going in the same direction as the original path. Maybe we needed to go through that processing all over again to join up some remaining dots that made clear which paths were appropriate and which were no longer needed.

Session 10 – 5 weeks later

Like many people, Cathy enjoyed the festive foods of Christmas but unlike many who use willpower to stop smoking and reduce their consumption of alcohol, she didn't find that party time caused her to want to smoke at all or drink any more than her recent normal amount – very little. That was really good news. She joined a gym and signed up for a 10k race. Once again, she describes the feeling as similar to when she was 11 years old. She's comfortable without cigarettes and alcohol, doesn't need them to have a good time and wouldn't dream of touching either. And her backache has improved even more since the previous session.

Once again, the treatment focussed on her gaining weight, and once again, all signs indicated that it had purely been due to the same underlying cause as the smoking, the dependence on alcohol, the backache and the excessive sweating. She had some loss of hearing which seemed to have started around the time she first started taking medication for depression, so we considered whether it could be a side effect of the tablets.

Session 11 – 5 weeks later

The gain in weight had stopped. Her weight had been stable since the previous session. There hadn't been any loss yet, but no gain either. Her backache continued to reduce but the hearing loss and buzzing in her ears were getting worse.

We focussed on her inability to lose weight and found that it was linked to another issue that had built up on the back of the original misunderstanding. Expressions like 'there's no smoke without fire' and 'give a dog a bad name' spring to mind here. In our judgements of other people and situations, we can assume that that purse was stolen by that same person who stole the sweets last year, but the sweet-toothed light-fingered youngster might have more recently grown up, learnt a lesson, developed a conscience and mended their ways.

Something like that can also happen within us, in the hidden depths of that part of the mind that decides who we are, what kind of person we will become and how such a person will live their life. Somewhere deep down inside us, far away from the light of day and more balanced and rational feedback from others, with all the best of intentions and with our best interests at heart, there could still be a miscarriage of justice.

An airline pilot will never wilfully or neglectfully allow the plane to crash, will always do their very best in all circumstances, will never give up trying while they are still breathing, because the fate of the pilot is exactly the same as that of the passengers, the crew, the aeroplane itself. They are all in the same situation.

Equally, the subconscious part of the mind sinks or swims, wins or loses, perishes or survives and even thrives side by side with the conscious mind and the body because it is our virtual conjoined twin.

But in spite of this alignment rather than conflict of interest, things still go wrong, planes still crash, people still have symptoms, conditions, issues that they don't want or need and can't get rid of.

Let's get back to Cathy. It seemed like all the information to resolve her inability to lose weight was already available to her subconscious mind, but there's no knowing how long it would have taken for that process to have completed if left to take place on its own, in the background. By walking that path together, the subconscious mind and I joined up the remaining dots and completed the picture so that remaining discomfort and unease, remaining symptoms and conditions could be wrapped up much more quickly and efficiently.

Again, time would tell.

Session 12 – 4 weeks later

Recently, Cathy had been, under medical supervision, reducing her anti-depressant dose, slowly and steadily, without any return of the depression. She was on the lowest dose and currently only taking it every other day.

Although there hadn't, as yet, been any reduction in her weight, she found that her eating habits and her cooking patterns had changed. Just like she went off the taste of cigarettes and alcohol, her taste for sweet and rich food was reducing.

Treatment, yet again, proved no further need for her to be unable to lose weight, and after the hypnosis, we discussed her return to exercise. She hadn't done much yet but was planning to start the Alexander Technique and as she has an interested and curious mind, maybe she needs a form of exercise where she is mentally as well as physically active.

Session 13 – 2 months later

She had some medical tests and received a diagnosis of an inner-ear disease that affects hearing and balance, and was happy to have had that confirmation.

She hadn't lost any weight, but no gain either. Her weight had been stable for about 4 months. Her appetite continued to reduce, so although she had been eating some rich, sweet food, she had eaten it in smaller quantities.

We treated what has been diagnosed as tinnitus, that she described as like a bee or wasp buzzing around her head, although clearly coming from inside, not outside of her.

We found another incident, and it was another one of those now inappropriate ones, the 'give a dog a bad name' ones, and her subconscious quickly reassessed it and added it to the to-do list of tidying up and recalibrating.

Session 14 – 2 months later

She had a further medical diagnosis around the hearing and dizziness, where she was told to expect it to only be temporary, which was much more reassuring.

We didn't do any treatment that day as the progress, to date, was so positive. Her weight had finally begun to reduce, very slowly and gradually going in the right direction. Her appetite and eating habits improvements had been maintained and she had been adding more exercise habits into her day and her week. She was going running and doing yoga, eating healthily with occasional treats. Her backache continued to improve, with no twinges since the last session and the dull ache virtually gone.

She was still enjoying being a non-smoker and a very light drinker and the embarrassing sweating was still gone. Her anti-depressant reduction continued without any return of the depression. That old once-familiar guilt and hyper-responsibility also continued to reduce.

The tinnitus and vertigo were still responding well to medication and she was expected to make a full recovery from both in time.

It didn't seem appropriate to do any further treatment. I concluded by asking her how she would feel about her story being one of the anonymous case studies in my second book, and she was happy to help me and my future clients in that way.

Chapter 7

Something we consider to be part of our character might be open to change

Pat: *So it wasn't exactly a simple smoking cessation treatment then?*

Me: No, that's right. I don't suppose any of my LCH colleagues would have done the single-session anti-smoking treatment in Cathy's case.

Chris: *That was in 2009 and 2010, but is she still not smoking?*

Me: I saw her in February 2011, had an email from her in September 2012 and saw her in July 2013. She's still not smoking. That's about 4 years now since that 'test' cigarette.

Chris: *I know people who gave up smoking decades ago and they still miss that one after a special meal. They still look a bit enviously at the gang of smokers outside the pub. They miss the social side of it all. Does Cathy feel like that?*

Pat: *I've never smoked a cigarette in my life, and I've never wanted to be part of a group of smokers, even many years ago when they could smoke whenever and wherever they wanted to. Do ex-smokers feel different from non-smokers?*

Me: I'm an ex-smoker, and I feel the same as you do, Pat, like a non-smoker. It seems that Cathy feels that way too, like she did when she was 11 years old. None of us has any urge to light up. Smoking doesn't feel like the solution to anything. It doesn't feel like a reward for a job well done, or a comfort in times of stress, or a treat on a special occasion. Cigarettes feel irrelevant. Urges and cravings and habitual reaching for the packet and the lighter are long gone and virtually forgotten for Cathy.

Chris: *And she seems to have got good value for the time and money she invested in all of those sessions. I think that, if that had been me, I would have felt very happy to have gained so much benefit in so many different aspects of my life in a matter of months.*

Me: From start to finish, it took a year, but most of the sessions were monthly.

And remember the discussion we had about what's likely to happen if someone has 2 or more addictions and the first one is treated and starts to reduce.

Chris: *Yes, that's right. I wasn't expecting to hear that a second addiction started to reduce when you'd only had chance to treat one of them. I would definitely have expected the other one to begin to increase, like when someone starts eating more when they stop smoking or smoking more when they go on a diet.*

Pat: *So I guess that's another indication that LCH works at the roots and those addictions had grown from the same set of roots or from the same inadvertently planted seed.*

So what did she say when you interviewed her? Was she happy with the results of her treatment?

Cathy's Thoughts - The interview – February 2011

Her experience of treatment

The process of treatment seemed to go smoothly for her. She knew she didn't need to play any conscious part in the problem-solving and was happy to leave her subconscious mind to do all the work. Some people are keen to know what it was all about but Cathy wasn't curious in the slightest. She was just happy to be feeling better.

She felt in safe hands and described the treatment and the hypnosis as gentle. She felt comfortable handing over control to her subconscious mind. She knew she was always able to take control back at any time.

It was actually a benefit to her that I wasn't prepared to provide single-session treatment because she had come to me a bit nervous of suddenly finding herself without her smoking habit. She didn't really know, on that first day, whether she was ready to let it go. It seemed a bit scary to manage without it.

Smoking

I remember you asked me what I expected to get out of the sessions and I said I wanted to feel as though I had never been a smoker. You said it wouldn't be possible to make me feel like that but in actual fact that is exactly how I do feel now!

Cathy didn't want to be a smoking grandma. She didn't want to be still smoking at 60.

We shared memories of days when smoking was regarded in a totally different way. People would smoke around children and even babies. When you worked in an office, people all around would be smoking without any awareness of the toxic fog they were creating for the non-smokers to breathe in.

The treatment worked 100%. She now wouldn't dream of having a cigarette, never in a million years.

She used to enjoy smoking. Initially, she didn't really want to give it up as she enjoyed the sensations and the relaxation, but knew that she needed to stop for the sake of her health. Now she wouldn't dream of lighting up a cigarette.

Cathy still doesn't want to smoke and now feels very much a non-smoker rather than an ex-smoker. She is totally in neutral around smokers now. She doesn't want or have any kind of urge to join them by having a cigarette. Equally, she doesn't feel any impatience or irritation towards those smokers either. If any of those smokers tell her they want to give up, she gives them my leaflet and recommends me and LCH.

She doesn't believe in quick fixes. She would always be wondering if that flicked switch would just as suddenly switch back again. Maybe that's why she felt a need to test it out.

She tried to smoke at her own party. She took a drag of a cigarette without any urge or craving, just a wish to see what would happen, to see if the addiction was gone completely or just hidden, lurking close by, waiting for a signal to come back. That first drag was unpleasant but she wanted to be sure, so she took another. That tasted worse but she wanted to be absolutely certain so she carried on with determination. After that third drag, she couldn't continue. She was finding it so unpleasant that she stubbed it out.

Many people have a cigarette weeks, months or years after giving up smoking, but then strangely find themselves back on the receiving end of that little voice suggesting that it's time for another cigarette. She didn't get that voice again, and to date, she never has. That party was in August 2009, and now, she is still happy because she doesn't have the slightest inclination to smoke.

Some people believe that nicotine is addictive, that it leaves its button there to be pressed by just one cigarette. In this case, for Cathy, it seems not to be have been the case.

I had a similar experience myself in that I spent years trying to give up and failing. Twice I became hooked again after just one cigarette when I'd enjoyed 6 months without. One day, when I was in my early 20's, suddenly, mysteriously, I just lost the taste for it. I found it unpleasant. I didn't even find myself drawn back to it when I was in great need of comfort.

A few months after the day that I lost the urge to smoke, my Mum died and grief almost overwhelmed me. It never crossed my mind to turn, even briefly, to cigarettes.

Before we found the cause, Cathy enjoyed smoking. After we found and resolved the cause, her taste for cigarettes and alcohol changed from enjoyment to dislike or even loathing. Her enjoyment of exercise has been rekindled after many years of not being able to get going. It just started to draw her interest and her enthusiasm again. She now enjoys running, yoga, Zumba and the gym.

She knows she used to smoke in the same way that she knows what playground games she played as a schoolgirl, and even though it's only about 3 years since she last smoked and more than 3 decades since she left school, they both seem equally distant memories now.

Pat: *Is the subconscious causing us to enjoy the things that it wants us to keep on doing?*

Chris: *That makes sense when you think of weird food cravings in pregnancy. They always seem to contain some kind of vitamin or mineral that the foetus probably needs for its development.*

Me: Yes, that makes sense to me too. The subconscious is always doing its best, and when it knows better, it does better.

That part of her mind that had previously told her how nice smoking felt now reminds her how awful cigarettes taste if anyone ever offers her one.

Drinking

When she came for treatment to stop smoking, she hadn't, at that time, had any real concern about how much alcohol she was drinking. She didn't mention it to me in the initial consultation. Looking back on it now, with a more distant and comfortable perspective, she can remember regularly drinking up to the point where, with just one more drink, she would have been likely to pass out. And then she would go to bed to wake up the next morning with an almighty hangover.

She hadn't seriously considered that it might have been a problem until she had found that she was beginning to enjoy a bright start to the day with no hangover. She only began to look at it that way when she started noticing that she was choosing healthier food and exercise to help unwind after a day at the office rather than several glasses of wine. She only saw the full extent of how it had been affecting her after she lost the automatic tendency to get to the point of one drink short of collapse. She only realised how much she had been suffering when she no longer woke up to a thumping head and a delicate stomach.

We never treated her alcohol habit. She didn't know she had a problem with it until, along with her previous urges and cravings to smoke, her urges to drink wine also started to reduce. By the time we'd made some progress with her smoking treatment, she was already finding herself going off the idea of drinking.

Cathy tested out the alcohol at a family gathering where she wanted to be sociable. She had never particularly wanted to stop drinking completely but when she found herself with no inclination to drink, had wondered if she had, in fact, had a drink problem. She wondered if she was free of it or if it was hiding, lurking in the background, waiting to take over again. She had a small glass of champagne for the toast and 2 small glasses of wine kept her going for the rest of the whole long social event of many hours.

The next morning she was extremely ill. She continued to feel ill for the rest of the day. She has had no urge to repeat that experience. I was concerned that that was taking away her choice. She reassured me that it is exactly what she wants. She enjoys the clear head, the clarity and refreshment of an evening without any fuzziness.

She especially enjoys the fact that she can go to bed knowing there will be no price to pay the next day. She treasures that sense of relief to know there will be no more hangovers - ever. She will feel good and be able to spend the day doing what she wants rather than restricted to whatever she can manage until the hangover slowly fades. It was the alcohol that had been taking away her choices. She feels much freer without it.

> *I had friends around for dinner and opened a bottle of Schloer apple juice, poured a glass and took a sip.................I had opened a bottle of red wine! I literally had to spit it out and pour the whole glass away, it was tantamount to me taking a sip of whiskey during my drinking days which I could never have done as I hate whiskey!*

She believes that the drinking could have ruined her life if it had carried on. She might easily have continued drinking more and more and the physical effects could have been extremely damaging.

Since the end of her treatment in the summer of 2010, she has come to know that she will spend the rest of her life as a teetotaller, knows that she will stay sober for ever and she feels good about it. She enjoys that clear head, that lack of fuzz, and especially enjoys waking up in the morning feeling refreshed and alert and healthy. She enjoys her social life without any feeling that something is missing.

Weight and Eating

She had lost 1 stone in about 3 months without dieting, without counting calories, without denying herself anything she wanted. From that point in her treatment when her weight started to increase, I had been concerned, but strangely, she had not been bothered by it. She had known it would be fine, that the weight would go again. Maybe some sixth sense or her subconscious was telling her that it was just a temporary phase, that it would sort itself out. It did!

Guilt and responsibility

Cathy had spent much of her life up to then with an ever-present sense that she was to blame for anything and everything that went wrong. Nearly 18 months later, she knows that she is doing her best. She is confident that her best is easily good enough. It no longer feels like the end of the world if things don't go to plan. It doesn't seem worth getting worked up about. She is much more comfortable with who she is and how she lives her life.

She describes her life as clearer now. She can see when she's getting tired. When she needs to rest, she rests, where in the past she would have battled on and then collapsed onto the settee at the end of the day with a drink and a smoke.

For many years, or even decades, she didn't treat herself because it felt wrong. It seemed selfish. She's a mum and the kids always came first. Having time to relax didn't feel right. She used to deny herself pleasures. Any time or money spent on herself felt like a luxury she couldn't afford and didn't deserve. She now finds healthy ways to reward herself when she believes she deserves a treat.

She had been keen to exercise many years ago, but when she had an ectopic pregnancy, she stopped it all and then never managed to pick it up again. But now she really enjoys it again. She has joined a gym, does yoga and goes running because she wants to. A 10k race is one of her recent achievements.

She eats when she wants to, eats what she wants to, takes more notice what kind of food she is putting in her mouth and is a lot fussier about it now. She used to just finish what was on her plate, but now stops when she's had enough. She still eats and still enjoys chocolate.

She had believed she needed cigarettes and alcohol to get through the day. She never used to give herself the luxury of a nap, and instead, would battle on through her tiredness, feeling selfish for wanting and needing a break or a rest.

Now, if she's had a particularly tiring day, she will have a cat nap or power nap rather than a drink or cigarette. Previously, she had needed one or both of those habits, alcohol and nicotine, to help her unwind after a stressful day, but now doesn't find herself feeling stressed in that way.

She doesn't feel like she's denying herself any pleasures, she doesn't feel deprived in any way. She can now enjoy a night out, have just as much fun, feel just as relaxed among friends, joining in the humour and banter when all she has had to drink all evening is soda water.

Since her last session with me in the summer of 2010, she bought herself an Aga cooker, something she had wanted for decades. Up to then, she hadn't found herself able to justify spending that much money on herself.

Now she sees rest and exercise, the gym and running, yoga and Zumba, healthy food and a stimulating social life as necessities she wouldn't dream of depriving herself of.

I use a lot of analogies in my explanations to my clients, and it must have rubbed off on Cathy. She came back with one of her own. She sees some treatments like power saws that chop off big branches, whereas LCH is like the JCB that digs up the unhealthy tree by the roots.

My thoughts

The process Cathy experienced with her smoking was probably like what happens when a minor cut or graze forms a scab. If we leave it alone, the scab will stay there until it's no longer needed. Once the skin underneath has knitted together and grown strong enough to survive without protection, the scab falls off and we might not even notice when it does. If we try to rush it and pick at the scab, it will hurt and bleed and form another scab. Cathy's urges to smoke fell away just like that scab because all the work underneath had been completed.

Maybe that's why a single session treatment felt so wrong to her. And maybe that's why the test cigarette left her so unmoved, unaffected. We don't find another scab forming after the first one simply fell off leaving strong and healthy skin underneath.

Sleep

I've heard that regular drinking can affect the quality of sleep. Some people who have come to me for treatment for insomnia have described their experience of taking prescribed sleep-medication. It can deliver a full night's sleep, not lying awake during the night, not tossing and turning, not worrying, not getting up in frustration as sleep won't come. The sufferer gets a full night's sleep but still wakes up as un-refreshed as if they'd had exactly that kind of disturbed and uncomfortable night.

I imagine that regular alcohol consumption can have that same effect, so a habit of going to bed on somewhere in the region of a bottle of wine could have left Cathy as tired and stressed out as an insomnia sufferer. So without that drinking habit, her sleep quality might have improved and helped her to cope. Work and all the other day to day events, frustrations, things not going to plan etc might have seemed less severe and more manageable than before so that she didn't need the previous habitual wind-down drink.

The Placebo effect

People talk about the Placebo effect in connection with all sorts of treatments and therapies. In traditional western medicine, it seems to be regarded as a nuisance that gets in the way of pure scientific pharmaceutical trials. Efforts are made to exclude people who seem to be most susceptible to Placebo. I have a much more positive opinion of the Placebo effect. Wherever it causes benefit, I believe we would benefit from studying it and learning more about it so we can help even more people to benefit.

But one essential component of Placebo is, by definition, that whatever the 'sugar pill' or other apparent intervention was, it was intended to benefit a particular condition. We wouldn't attribute benefits to some other condition, something that wasn't being studied, as Placebo effect.

It seems like Cathy's subconscious detected the connection between the cause of the smoking habit and need for the drinking, the guilt and the sweating, and went on ahead to do some overtime, above and beyond the work Cathy and I were asking for.

The only explanation I can offer as to why her drinking, her excessive and embarrassing sweating and her underlying sense of guilt all mysteriously disappeared once we found the cause of her smoking was that they were linked at the roots and her subconscious did a great and thorough job.

Our thoughts

As we drew the interview to a close, we found ourselves discussing whether other groups of people might benefit from LCH. Some people with a severe drug addiction resort to crime to finance their habit. Maybe some of those would choose a more socially benign and legal lifestyle that was better for them, for their potential victims and for society, if LCH could be employed to unlock the door of their cell of crack cocaine or heroin habit.

Maybe there are some who, however hard they try to drag themselves up from the depths, find that something, some unknown, hidden, mysterious internal force always seems to drag them back down. Maybe some of those people could be helped by LCH. Maybe someone who works in a relevant field will read this and consider researching into the wider possibilities of LCH.

Extracts from recent emails from Cathy

September 2012

> ... *you've given me a new perspective on life and I feel so much better than I did eighteen months ago....*

> *...I'm always telling people about you, they're fascinated to learn how I was able to stop smoking AND drinking! ... I would be more than happy to help you out with your second book....*

November 2012

> *After a rather nasty cold and not wanting to drink coffee, I have not touched coffee since! I used to live on the stuff to get some energy!*

I needed to know more, so emailed back this request for more information: -

Would you tell me a bit more about this, please? e.g. Before that cold, if you didn't drink coffee or couldn't get enough, were you very tired? Did you suffer any withdrawal when you had that cold? How do you feel now, after that further change in your habits? Have you found yourself caffeine free or do you have tea and/or drinks like cola? What are your energy levels like now? etc. etc.

> *... I never liked coffee in my teens and early twenties and when I did start drinking it, drank very little, went right off it with each pregnancy and I think only really started enjoying it mid thirties. When I started smoking again at 42, coffee and cigarettes went hand in hand and it was often a case of having a coffee so that I could have a cigarette.*
>
> *Before the smoking ban, working in hotels meant that coffee was always 'on tap' and I did tend to live on caffeine and nicotine to get some energy. I have felt extremely and constantly tired for the past ten years which I now feel may be something to do with the underactive thyroid that has just been diagnosed. Apparently, it can progress over a number of years and once thyroid levels have dropped to a figure that doctors are able to medicate for, the thyroid gland has actually stopped producing thyroxin completely.*
>
> *So yes, I drank coffee to get some energy. However, I didn't get any withdrawal symptoms at all. In the*

*past when I've cut down my coffee consumption,
I've experienced horrible headaches but not this
time. I do still drink tea but no fizzy drinks.*

*I am struggling quite badly with energy levels,
I've been on Levothyroxin for a couple of months
but only a small dose which is being monitored
monthly until I am at the right levels. Apparently,
it's important to start off slowly as an initial high
dose can cause a stroke!*

*I'm hoping that the malaise I've been feeling
will be alleviated by the medication although
I'm not expecting a quick fix. Also, I think that
my weight gain has been partially caused by this
Hypothyroidism and am looking forward to a
turnaround there too.*

July 2013

**Following on from a discussion we had in early
July, where Cathy was happy to tell me of yet more
changes she believes she is enjoying because of the
treatment that 'keeps on giving', she offered to write
up one of those developments for me.**

*When I was thirteen my parents separated. My father
left home and the 'marital' home was sold. When I was
fifteen my mother remarried and we moved twenty
miles out into the country to do up an old cottage.
I carried on attending my old school and caught a bus
which meant a two hour journey each day.*

*I found it hard to move away from friends,
particularly as I had been dating for the past few
months. I was very lonely each evening, during
weekends and holidays. I couldn't afford the bus
fares to go back to my old village and of course
couldn't drive.*

*I spent a lot of time in my room, reading and
listening to music. One of the songs that became a
particular tearjerker was Puppy Love by Donny
Osmond. Some songs continue to stir emotion years
later and whenever I heard this song it would stop
me in my tracks and all the emotions from that time
would come flooding back.*

*It got to the point where I would turn the radio
off when it came on. However, recently I was
listening to an edition of 'Pick of the Pops' when
I heard the first few bars of Puppy Love and
thought I was in for another emotional reminder.
To my surprise, there was no physical or mental
reaction at all, I waited, expecting to feel the same
tug on the heartstrings, but nothing. I played it
again recently and can honestly say that I don't
think it's ever going to have the same effect on
me again.*

There has been some more treatment since the latest
described above, and this is the latest pre-publication
update on her response to that treatment. Any further
updates, where appropriate, will be outlined in my
third book.

September 2013

I can't thank you enough for your help in changing my life. If I hadn't picked up your card that day I would very possibly not be here now, my life was really spiralling out of control and I had no way of knowing how to get it back. I would never have seeked help for my drinking, I didn't even consider it a problem but looking back it certainly was. Maybe something pushed me to come to you for that reason and not for the smoking.......maybe that was a 'smokescreen' (pardon the pun!).

Over the past six months I've reflected on some of the things which I feel shouldn't have happened in my life, things which I let happen, things which other people would have refused to put up with and I've made a decision to say 'no' when I want to. To be a bit more selfish and not to agree to everything that's asked of me. At 54 soon to be 55 I think I've earned the right to live my life how I want to now. I can only think that my subconscious is suggesting a 'better way' now.

*I'm arranging an appointment to have my thyroid levels checked and once I know the results I'll email you. Also, am very nearly off the anti-depressants :) just take a half one every three days. This is after fifteen years of the b***** things!!*

I'm so glad to be living proof that there can be an alternative to years of medicine and therapy.

Pat and I discuss single-session again

Pat: *So was that anti-smoking treatment exactly like the way you treat any other symptom, or did you create a mixture of the 2 approaches?*

Me: We never worked directly on the smoking habit itself. I never gave a single instruction during hypnosis about not smoking, not wanting to smoke, not having any urges or cravings. The only instructions I gave were to help her relax and respond to treatment so that I could work with her subconscious mind to uncover and resolve the underlying cause. It was purely LCH.

Pat: *So has that treatment affected your assessment of single-session treatment versus LCH. I imagine you have more confidence in your decision now.*

Me: Yes, it feels like the safest way to proceed. I know that a single-session therapy works for many people, but there are others, like Cathy, for whom a slower process feels more natural and comfortable, thorough and appropriate.

Pat: *What do you think would have happened if you had done a single-session treatment?*

Me: I believe that, if I had treated her smoking using direct suggestion, then she might have easily stopped smoking and then have found herself drinking even more. I think that whatever was at the root of her smoking habit must have also been at the root of her drinking as well.

Pat: *So do you think I should focus only on LCH treatment once I've qualified?*

Me: No, I believe you should listen to the arguments for and against and then make up your own mind. I think you should do the same as I do after that, which is continue to do what feels right to you and continue to consider any new arguments you hear. Then, if you find the pros and cons end up balanced in the opposite direction, adjust your work in line with what seems right to you.

Chris and Pat and I discuss what benefits are possible with LCH

Chris: *I was thinking about all of that stuff about her feeling responsible and feeling guilty. I have some of that too, and until you told me about Cathy, I always thought that that kind of thing was part of a person's personality. When I think about people that I know, I'd say that some of them are like me in that they are always somehow driven to put other people's needs first. They struggle to say no even when they're overloaded.*

Pat: *I agree, and I can't imagine many people thinking about hypnotherapy for conditions like that. Have you had anyone come to you for treatment for anything along those lines?*

Me: Not that I can remember. I've mainly seen people gain benefits in that kind of way when they've come to me for something else, like an unrelated habit or phobia.

Chris: *Hmmm... food for thought for me, then....*

Me: Pat and Chris, what are the main messages for you from this case?

Pat: *I think the confirmation that LCH works at the roots is reassuring. It's easy to imagine that a second or third addiction might have the same cause and might be serving the same subconscious purpose. I can't think of any other explanation for why the alcohol and caffeine habits went away when you never even treated them.*

Chris: *For me, the main idea is that something we might consider to be part of our character or personality, like always feeling guilty and responsible for the feelings of others, is something that might actually be open to change. That could be a huge relief for many people. If people know that there is the chance they can get help that could bring long-lasting change, I'm sure many would want to hear more about it and maybe give it a try.*

Chapter 8

Please don't expect me to be anything other than at least a little bit contrary

Chris: *I'd like to know a bit more about how you came to be a therapist. You've mentioned, a few times, that you used to be a computer programmer. That sounds like a huge leap in the dark to retrain in hypnotherapy.*

Pat: *Tell us a bit more about what led up to you changing career and how the first few years were for you. I'm still feeling a bit unsure about whether it's right for me and whether I'm right for it. Your experience might help me decide.*

Me: It might help, Pat, but you also need to remember that we all approach things in our own way and we all progress differently, and with a name like 'Mary', please don't expect me to be anything other than at least a little bit contrary.

Also, as I explained briefly in 'What if...', along the way, I had treatment for various issues of my

own, including my lack of self-confidence, my
lack of belief in my ability to succeed, maybe
even a fear of success that probably sabotaged or
hampered some of my LCH development.

This really is just how it was for me.

Pat: Ok, I understand.

Several years ago, some time in 2004, I found myself
in a worrying situation. I had a well-paid job doing
something I liked and that stimulated that problem-
solving part of my mind/brain – and then they told me,
'you'd better review your C.V.' I had survived numerous
restructuring and downsizing phases in my company
and had developed a calm and confident assumption
that it would never affect me. Then I heard someone say
that restructuring, downsizing and offshore outsourcing
were endemic. There was no way I would escape forever.

But I had no 'plan B' and I felt exposed.

Then some of those strange life-event nudges, that we
can choose to ignore or be steered by, seemed to be
sending me in a particular direction. I had always
had an interest in matters relating to the mind. My
work-experience included several years in the caring
profession specialising in mental health. Psychology
fascinated me. Hypnosis and hypnotherapy sounded
intriguing and I wanted to know more.

Someone I knew was planning on giving up smoking.
At the time, I was investing some of my leisure time on
Reiki. I had trained in Reiki I and II and was treating

friends and family whenever given half a chance.
I offered to give my friend a Reiki treatment, which he
seemed pleased to accept and found the experience
enjoyable and relaxing. He also had hypnotherapy from
a neighbour and is now happy to be a non-smoker.

Nudge number 1 was when I asked for some information
from the hypnotherapist who had treated my ex-smoker
friend about the training he had had. The response came
back in the form of a prospectus for a hypnotherapy
training establishment in a town where an acquaintance
of mine lived.

Nudge number 2 came from my acquaintance of whom
I asked, 'Do you know of this training college in your
town?' The reply was something like 'No but if you
want to train in an advanced form of hypnotherapy
that achieves lasting results, then you need to check
out these guys'. He handed me the business card of a
therapist and I set off to follow some clues.

Various phone calls and internet searches later, my
mind was buzzing with interest and enthusiasm.
I found the website of the highly-recommended
training college and got myself some reading material
which led me to have some treatment for my own
conditions and issues, and to enrol on the initial stage
of the training program.

This started with a correspondence course, the Home
Study. It involved a number of modules where questions
were posed and you were invited to think, to let your
enquiring instincts take you beyond any existing

knowledge you might have – and to respond with whatever was the best you could come up with based on your own reasoning, common sense, logical thought and experience. I was in my element. There was no right or wrong – as long as you could explain, step by step, how you came to any of your responses, then that was all that was being asked of you.

I completed all the modules to the satisfaction of the College and enrolled for the next stage. I paid a fairly substantial sum of money with a quiet inner knowledge that this was money that I was meant to spend. I had always lived within my means to satisfy my huge need for financial security and from some kind of intuition that 'knew' that one day, there would be something so worthwhile that I would want and need to invest in it.

The next stage was the Practical Course. There were eight attendees, the tutor and a teaching assistant. The attendees were made up of one person who had done the course a few years before but hadn't gone into practice, so his skills had lapsed. He was attending it as a refresher. One person was already a hypnotherapist and wished to extend her knowledge and skills and effectiveness, and the remaining 6 people, including myself, were totally new to any kind of hypnotherapy including Lesserian™ Curative Hypnotherapy.

The Practical Course was composed of 5 weekends of theory, practice and of observing the treatment of 3 volunteer clients. The tutor explained some theory and I asked quite a few questions. I wasn't the only one to ask, but I was the one who asked the most.

Apparently, there's nearly always someone on each
course who fits that role, and it was me that time.
It wasn't long before the tutor was turning to me
at the end of each "and does anyone have any
questions....Mary?"

Once again, I was in my element. My questions were
getting answered in plain English, no jargon to hide or
blur the messages, and the information, on the whole,
made sense to me. I was being encouraged to explore
any ambiguities, to ask the 'yes, but...' questions. And
as time went on, my mind and my questions started to
go off at various tangents which meant that the tutor
had 'not been asked that one before'. Her response to
some of those situations was to take the question away
with her and come back later with something that filled
in the gap, that explained where I had missed some
vital link or misunderstood some idea or concept.

More recently, I'm still asking those 'yes, but...'
questions, and often find that I haven't missed or
misunderstood anything. It's just that there is more
than one way, more than one path to follow, and
sometimes my path is different from my tutor's path –
but just as valid and similarly therapeutically effective.
And we both believe that diversity is so important to
the development of strong theories, robust techniques,
safe methods, so we often discuss our differing views in
order to dig deeper, learn more, continuously improve
what we do and how we do it.

Back to 2006. 3 volunteer clients were being treated in
front of us. There were theories to study and analyse,

practical techniques to learn, a written exam and a viva. I passed.

> Clutching my certificate, I needed to convert all of that training into a hypnotherapy practice where I gained results, where I gave my clients good value, where the hope and time and money they invested in their treatment was more than returned by the improvement in the quality of life they achieved.

I set off...

But I felt very similar to the way I felt when I first got behind the wheel of my own car, wondering how on earth I had convinced the examiner to give me my driving licence, and how I was going to drive without someone 'holding my hand'. Having spoken to some other people in similar circumstances since then, it seems I wasn't alone – but it felt that way at the time.

So I decided to behave like a walker, up on the hills, not much of a map-reader but with a few clues, a whole heap of motivation and a dogged determination to get there, even if it meant one small step at a time, and even if that 'step' was down a steep and slippery slope that was so scary that the best I could do was sit down and shuffle along on my bottom, with hands and feet clutching at any clump of grass to slow down my descent.

My tutor, Helen Lesser, may have been amazed at such graphic descriptions. She has somewhere in the region of

30 years of experience around this therapy. Her father, David Lesser, laid the foundation stones, believed totally in its effectiveness, and worked tirelessly towards achieving even more of what he knew could result from successful analytical problem-solving hypnotherapy treatment.

Helen attended his training course and then worked alongside him, absorbing all he was able to teach her and then asking herself some 'yes, but' questions in order to take the treatment forwards to where it became even more effective, the results even more reliable and long-lasting. As a result, she had added some vital floors to the building, some essential rooms to those floors so that what her father had designed and initiated could be shared even more with others, could be passed on even more thoroughly in training.

She worked, and still works, constantly and conscientiously towards adding more and more functionality and efficiency to the whole process - and has many very happy, much relieved ex-clients who are now living more comfortable and healthy lives as a result of her work – the ex-clients she has treated herself and also those treated by the therapists who have successfully completed her training courses.

She has continued the work her father started in 1978 of passing on these powerful techniques, these compelling theories – and since his death in 2001, has run the training college and once or twice a year sent some newly qualified therapists out into various parts of the country to begin their incredible journey.

Looking back to the job I had in 2004, for nearly 20 years, I had been a computer programmer. It requires a kind of problem-solving logic to come naturally, or the potential for it to develop. It also requires a belief that, if something is going wrong in a program, if it's not completing - or it is, but the results make no sense, or there's some strange and indecipherable error message appearing, then **there has to be a reason.**

Ok, there has to be a reason, but, at least going back to my early days as a programmer, that reason could be a single line of code anywhere in hundreds, thousands or even tens of thousands of lines. It could be wrong in itself, or it could be a valid line in the wrong place.

So much of the explanation I heard on the hypnotherapy course made the same kind of sense. Something, some incident, some event, some information, some experience from some time in the client's life could be wrong, or in the wrong place. But forget hundreds, thousands and tens of thousands. We're talking so many noughts on the end that there isn't an '...illions' kind of name for it.

Imagine a multi-sensory recorder, a video recorder that adds in touch, taste and smell, recording every single experience that the client has had since time for them began – whether we believe that is the moment of birth, the moment of conception, or somewhere in between (or from some previous life – depending on our belief system), who knows. It records the raw data, the sensory input, the sounds, the sights, the physical feelings, all the emotional reactions to that data - and all the interpretations of all of that, made at the time and revised at any other time.

And something in all that, one tiny detail in all that, is that wrong or misplaced line of code!

I had spent nearly 20 years defying the odds and finding rogue lines of code in computer programs, and getting better at it. Columbo, that wonderful fictional TV detective who kept me entertained and amused on so many a rainy weekend afternoon, was my hero. I started learning how to follow clues, how to narrow down my search, how to look beyond the obvious, to dismiss whole chunks of the program because some tiny detail I'd found confirmed that they couldn't contain the error.

So I knew it was possible, and I knew I had the kind of problem-solving logic and the interest in using those skills, that even after nearly 20 years at a computer screen, could get me saying 'Is it 5 o'clock already? I must have got engrossed!'

As soon as I was given my Certificate, I started putting the various building blocks in place, one by one – and from that narrow ledge high up in the hills, on that misty winter's afternoon when the light was fading and civilisation seemed such a long way away, when the destination was totally out of sight, I didn't look down. I didn't dare!

I started by joining a couple of professional organisations and getting myself the vital professional indemnity insurance. I reviewed my notes, looked at what I needed to do and realised how unprepared I felt for the task ahead. I had various scripts that I'd been given for standard CDs to give to clients to help in the progress of treatment. Several attempts at using different techniques to record them led eventually to something I felt I could at least make some kind of start with.

One of the recording methods I discarded along the way was a fairly cheap microphone which was not very sensitive. I found myself, at some late hour in the evening, saying, in the loudest projection I could manage, "1... SLEEP, 2... SLEEP, ... AND YOU ARE BECOMING MORE AND MORE RELAXED AND COMFORTABLE..." I wonder what my neighbour must have thought as she went to her doorway to call in her cats.

I soon learnt that after 10pm in the back bedroom with all phones switched off was the best way to avoid getting 18 minutes into a 20 minute script only to have someone knock on the door and try to sell me cable TV, ask me who supplies my gas and electricity or talk to me about my eternal salvation.

It seemed like I had to find a way to actually get started

I didn't have much idea but thought I'd try finding someone to practise on, if there was anyone brave or daft enough to put their life – or mind – in my hands. My first 'volunteer' allowed me to do a consultation and an initial hypnosis session and then politely but firmly declined to go beyond that. My second attempt went a bit further. She allowed me to take one manageable step at a time.

So I had one client. I was insured. I had letters after my name and a reputable organisation behind me, and I had one CD and a pretty good idea how to do session 1. I'd already done that one. I felt almost experienced.

So from then on, I worked in a kind of 'hand to mouth' or 'just in time' way, preparing each session and each CD just prior to delivering them. It was all I could manage. Any more than that and I felt like I was staring across that ravine with no idea how I would get to the other side.

And as far as I could tell, it all went fairly well. The universe had been kind to me. My practice client was a textbook case who responded like a dream. So I thought I knew it all. I thought I'd got the hang of it and just needed to get a bit better, a bit quicker. I was wrong. I had so much to learn. Textbook cases are few and far between and people can and do respond in so many different ways that I needed to learn more and more about.

As I started to treat my clients, on a part-time basis, while still in full-time employment as a computer programmer, I had taken the College's advice and started working on the 9-module Diploma course to advance towards full qualification. I started to learn some of the finer points I'd missed. I needed to work on them and fine-tune them before my clients could gain the level of benefit that I aimed to give them.

But just like the new driver, once that test is passed, as wrong as it feels, the only way to proceed, the only way to become an experienced and competent driver, is to get behind the wheel and take as much care as possible, be as cautious as necessary to avoid causing any harm while learning that competence.

I designed and printed leaflets and spent many happy Saturdays wandering round the city centre and neighbouring areas putting them in waiting rooms in hairdressers, nail and tanning studios, barbers, doctors, dentists and anywhere else where people might sit and get so bored they'd read anything.

I rented a room on an hourly basis and started out with a 4-hour slot on a Sunday afternoon where I often found myself with 1 or 2 clients and the occasional sad day with no-one at all. It was the sad feeling on those days that prompted me to get some professional help in designing and creating my website.

Maybe the universe was being kind again, but I bumped into an ex-colleague who helped put together a website. Without much input from me it totally fitted my personality and the message I wanted to send out to potential clients. People tell me that they found my site, amongst the several that they checked out, to be the one that resonated with them and led them to pick up the phone.

Those sad days, of sitting and waiting with no-one getting in touch, began to reduce steadily once the website was up and running and easily found by the most well-known search engines.

And I worked and worked and worked. I treated my clients and most got some benefit, but I knew that I could help them even more and I wasn't going to rest until I felt there was nothing else I needed to learn. I'm not expecting to ever get to that point. There's always room for improvement, so I don't need any kind of pressure on me to complete the required number of hours a year of Continued Professional Development (CPD). It just comes naturally to keep on studying, analysing and researching.

I was still doing the day job and spent most evenings preparing for my treatments, drafting another submission of the current Diploma module, reading through old journals and e-group messages for clues to help me get better at treating more people, to help them get more benefit from fewer sessions.

With each Diploma module, I found something else that I hadn't fully grasped or where I had gone off at a tangent, and with a childish optimism assumed that that would be enough for me to get the kind of results I craved and that I believed my clients deserved and had a right to expect from me.

And by the summer of 2007, it felt like I needed to do more.

I felt very unhappy about it all but wasn't anywhere near considering giving up my quest or sinking in to complacency. I just knew I had the skills required and that the treatment that I had sweated over was capable of delivering its promise of lasting, even permanent, benefits.

I needed help and decided the best plan was to redo the Practical Course as a refresher. It was a lot cheaper than the first time around and anyway, I still had the day job with a half-decent salary to fund it with. I knew that I would be able to take in some of the information that I'd missed the first time around.

I presented my anonymised notes to my tutor who went through them with her characteristic attention to detail. She found very little that was wrong or missing or muddled. She gave me some ideas to help with one of my current clients and the refresher course gave me loads of confirmation of huge chunks that I did know, that I had understood.

By that time I was on Module 5 of the Diploma and a couple more gaps had just been pointed out to me.

In some cases, I learned later that my memory of the treatments was biased towards the negative. I was having more success than I perceived. I saw anything less than a 100% complete and permanent cure after just a very small number of sessions as having been a total failure but in fact, more of my clients were gaining some degree of relief. Some were giving up treatment because their hopes and expectations of some improvement had already been met and they weren't aware that more would have been possible if they had continued their treatment.

Right from the start, I knew enough not to do any harm and most of my clients were going away with some degree of improvement. And even those few who gained no relief from their symptoms had a relaxing experience and gained some insight into the workings of the subconscious mind. They hadn't been taking pills with possible side effects. They hadn't had any kind of surgery with a risky anaesthetic. They had just got very relaxed and been asked some questions designed to solve problems, fix symptoms, resolve issues.

I occasionally get messages, many months and even years after treatment, that tell me of some continued improvement that I had helped start off without even knowing that I had. I bump into someone in a shop and they smile with recognition and happily report that things are still improving, or I get the same kind of information from a new client who passes on that kind of feedback from the person who highly recommended me.

I was (and still am) always aiming for the 'happily ever after', so on the journey towards that, I often found myself crossing treatments off as failures just because they weren't 100% totally, permanently, verifiably successful.

During those early years, I never gave up or even considered it. I was still working at the day job and spending time, energy and money on becoming a more effective therapist. And I did that because life's been good to me. I'd like to share some of what's overflowing from my much more than half full glass because I know there are loads of people living with pain and worry and progressively worsening conditions that medical science has had to reluctantly give up on, because I believe there's an answer for many of these people in Lesserian™ Curative Hypnotherapy, and because my mind is like that border collie eagerly looking for the next challenge as long as it's interesting and stretches my problem-solving skills.

At the end of 2007, I was made redundant from my programming job, given a handshake filled with enough financial security to send me on my way with few of the real-life worries and constraints that were causing others to tread cautiously.

Since then, I successfully completed the Diploma and treated lots of clients, and all of that time and energy and analysis has brought me to where I am now. Some of those people have told me that I helped to make a significant positive difference to their lives.

I think the best way I can deliver even more successful LCH therapy is to think, think and think some more, to enjoy thinking, to find it stimulating, challenging, intriguing to not know exactly where I'm going but just have an ever-growing belief that

**I have all I need inside me to get there even if
I couldn't see much of it when I first set off.**

Chris: *Thank you. That was all very interesting and
it's clear to me how much you've put into it.*

Pat: *I agree, but I'm not sure you've persuaded me
to start the training. There were quite a few
examples here where you didn't do things that
well and didn't seem confident in your abilities.
You needed to redo the Practical Course, too,
so is the course not possible to absorb all in
one go?*

Me: Pat, I don't want to persuade you or anyone
else to start training. I want to give you as clear
and as honest an account as I can. One very
important detail I need to remind you of is that
I needed treatment for a subconscious barrier I
had getting in the way of me being successful.
I clearly didn't know it was there until I'd
gone a fair way into the training and further
development. That is likely to be quite rare, to
have such a barrier – not unique but quite rare.

I want you to make up your own mind. This
isn't a marketing brochure. I'm not trying to
drum up business for the College. If people
decide to start the training having read my
story, then my aim is that they only train if it's
right for them.

The Practical Course is very intensive, but
repeating it isn't needed by everyone. I believe
we all need to work in our own way towards

becoming the kind of therapist and delivering the standard of treatment that our clients need and deserve from us. Some of us get nearer and nearer to that standard with, and some without, repeating the Practical Course. Some get all they need from the Diploma. Others work with more experienced colleagues, receiving supervision, coaching, mentoring.

I also think it's a powerful message that we learn as we wobble, that it's important to pick ourselves up when we fall, that we need to have the will and determination to keep going, and that, if we keep going, then wonderful things happen for the people we treat.

Pat: *Well you've certainly got across that the course and the subsequent work involves a certain kind of inquiring mind, motivation, being prepared to put time and effort into it, and if some of the hurdles you had to get over were due to your own individual 'barrier', then it sounds manageable to me.*

Chris, what do you think about Mary's warts and all account? Has it affected your decision about whether to go to her for treatment?

Chris: *If there had been success after success right from the start, all the things that went well and nothing else, I would have known that that couldn't have been the true story. Life isn't like that. I would have known I was being given a glossy, air-brushed, well spun tale and would have known that darker stories had been left untold.*

If someone tells me they are taking seriously and thoroughly examines any 'near misses', then I feel safer than if they assure me that everything is perfect, always was and always will be.

If something sounds too good to be true, it probably is. This sounds like real life and that makes me feel safe. Look at the medical profession and how many times the doctors and scientists have discovered that a well-meaning treatment was doing more harm than good. Thalidomide to cure morning sickness caused severe birth defects. Prolonged bed rest after an operation led to deep vein thrombosis. Amphetamines were, in my lifetime, routinely prescribed as slimming tablets.

Our health professionals always were, are, and always will be doing their best, always diligent, always watching and analysing and quickly correcting any adverse and unintended consequences. I still go to the doctor when I need to in spite of what has occurred throughout medical history because I know how many safeguards are in place.

I have a friend who is an athlete and she described to me once that, as she was going through her development, she had to work especially hard to achieve what some others sailed through. They had the right physique for their particular sport - and she didn't. Later on, though, when they all moved from the junior leagues to the adult ones and competed with the best in the country, some of those who had had the most physical advantages had no mental resilience to work and persevere and struggle.

They pretty soon gave up, but she found it much easier to apply herself, deal with setbacks, work on alternative strategies and make small but steady steps in the right direction. She believes that that early need to struggle is a powerful force that helps us rather than hinders us as we strive to reach our goals.

I feel safe knowing that Mary had some lessons to learn and some issues to resolve. I believe that going through all of that has probably contributed to her individual style. There are bound to be far more than the people written about here who are very grateful to her for not giving up, for not being complacent and cavalier about her clients' time and money and precious hopes for relief.

Pat: *Hmmm... That's certainly a perspective I hadn't thought of.*

And as for my decision about training, I was all excited about signing up for the course and felt disappointed hearing about some of Mary's 'wobbles' along the way. But now I'm going to take some more time. I don't want to make a decision on adrenaline. I want to make my mind up when it's right for me.

CHAPTER 9

There was just one tiny detail getting in his way

Pat: *You've told us about two clients where they needed quite a number of sessions. Is that always how it is? Do people need to expect that treatment will take a long time and sometimes have wide-spread ramifications? Can you tell us about one that didn't take quite so many sessions now?*

Chris: *Yes, I agree. It would be good to hear about a treatment that was completed quite quickly and didn't send ripples out into the person's life in a more general way.*

Me: That's fine. The person who came to me to stop nail-biting had that kind of experience. We only needed 5 sessions altogether. There's very little about the 'before and after' story that is remarkable in any way. He came to me for treatment and by the end of those 5 sessions, his habit had gone and to date, hasn't returned.

Pat: *Did you have any particular reason for choosing to include this person's treatment?*

Me: Yes, there was an aspect of it that made me particularly keen to include this account. There was a fairly unusual response to the treatment process from this person, a response that surprised me as well as him. In something like 7 years of practice, I've not seen anything quite like this and we both thought it had an impact all of its own.

Steve is a business man and a family man, highly motivated to succeed, to support himself and his family. He is confident in his own abilities, his skills, his creativity, his energy and drive. He is proud of his achievements and is keen to be the best he can be, to create the best business he can. He has a logical mind and as a problem-solver, is prepared to use his own skills and learn from others to improve, to make progress and develop further.

He consistently aims to satisfy his customers and create a good and secure income for himself, his family and his employees. He has a good social life, is physically fit and healthy, active, sporty, regularly working out at the gym.

But, and clearly there just has to be a 'but', there was just one tiny detail getting in his way, holding him back, hampering his progress. It had been on his mind for a while that this tiny 'fly in the ointment' has overstayed its welcome. It was long overdue for removal. He needed to find a solution. He had tried everything he could think of but that hadn't produced a long-term solution, just some brief periods of relief that had taken a lot of effort to maintain. He was keen to get it properly fixed and was open to getting help from a professional if necessary.

That was a brief picture of how things were for him when we met at a networking event in late 2009. We discussed our own and each other's businesses, and pretty soon, I detected some signs of personal interest and gave him a leaflet. I suggested he rang me if he wanted to discuss it further.

He'd seen stage hypnosis, had stayed firmly in his seat, had enjoyed the show but had had no urge to volunteer. He didn't know of anyone, a friend or relative or colleague, who had had hypnotherapy, so he hadn't had the benefit of hearing about it from someone he knew and trusted. He knew that hypnotherapy was bound to be different from stage hypnosis, but wasn't sure exactly in what way.

He hadn't been actively seeking a solution when he met me, but it had been lurking in the back of his mind. It was permanently on his 'getting around to it' list. He knew he wanted to give it a go – but had to wait for the right time, the right circumstances. Some time in early spring 2010, late February, early March, he got in touch and booked an initial session.

Chapter 10

The subconscious mind
is invited to work with me,
to do some remedial work

Session 1

I invited Steve to fill me in on the details of what he
wanted to have treatment for. He would bite his nails
and any loose skin on his fingers and his knuckles.
He mainly did it absent-mindedly. The first thing he
noticed was when he heard that inevitable click as teeth
meet and worse still, that sickening sting of broken
or torn skin and the occasional sight of drawn blood.
He had expected to grow out of it, but instead, had
become accustomed to it. As an adult, he wanted rid of
this habit as it was affecting his business as well as his
self-confidence. He expected people to react with a
'ugh' feeling.

He had done it as long as he could remember, although
in the early years, he never really gave it a thought
because it wasn't that unusual a habit for a child. It
happened most when he was under stress. His business
involves working to deadlines, writing, creating, looking

for ideas and inspiration. He would sit at his computer, one hand on the mouse, other hand, fingers in mouth. It also happened as he watched his team playing rugby. The more stressed he was feeling, the tighter the deadlines, the more intensely he would bite and pick at his nails and hands, but it was always there to some degree, in the background. It never fully went away.

He felt puzzled, confused and concerned about this habit usually associated with children, normally grown out of. It made his hands look unprofessional. He has to give demonstrations to prospective and current clients. He needs to point out details, which causes his hands, and especially his nails, to be on show. He wants and needs his hands to look well-cared-for. It's just like wearing a smart suit, keeping his hair well-groomed, driving a good-quality car. He needs to show himself in a good light to inspire confidence that he is running a business that is successful because it's good at what it does and delivers what it promises.

Clients need to feel safe to enter into contracts with him. He believes that bitten nails can give an impression of nervousness, lack of confidence, maybe even give a false impression that the business is in trouble. As he would bite his nails absent-mindedly, his clients and prospective customers might have not just seen the effects of his habit. They might have actually seen him biting in the middle of a progress demonstration or sales pitch.

When it first started to bother him, when he first noticed that it wasn't going to be good for business, he tried various measures to deal with it himself.

He started with willpower. He made a determined effort to stop biting, but it just kept happening before he noticed what he was doing, before he had chance to decide not to. He didn't even notice his hands go towards his mouth. By the time he noticed, it was always too late. Another chunk of nail had been at least partially detached.

He tried nurturing one nail at a time. He decided on one nail to look after and tried to make sure he left that one alone when biting. He focussed the habit totally on the other 9 until he could see the beginnings of a strong, sound, attractive nail beginning to develop. The sight of that nail was a bit of an incentive. The availability of other nails to feed the urges to bite helped him stick to his plan of removing his habit from each nail in turn. But it didn't last long. His final objective of all 10 nails intact and well-cared for wasn't reached that way either.

He used that nasty-tasting varnish that you paint on. It's supposed to taste so awful that you find it difficult to continue biting. He found himself getting used to the taste and then simply forgetting to paint it on.

Everything he tried worked for a little while, but took so much energy and motivation to maintain, so eventually, inevitably, he found himself slipping back into his habit – and getting more and more annoyed and frustrated with himself.

He wanted to have hands that looked the part - that fitted his professional image. He intended to get a manicure as soon as he had managed to stop biting.

He had a major contract to bid for in a few months' time and especially wanted this resolved by then so that he could give himself the best chance of winning it. He didn't want the state of his nails to tip the balance against any contract he would otherwise have won.

He expected that hypnotherapy would help him develop increased willpower so that he would be more able to control his habit.

The measures he had tried before coming to see me could be compared to bailing out the water from a leaking boat. This would inevitably need to continue, on and on, if the water was coming from a hole in the bottom of the boat. LCH could be related to the process of finding and fixing the hole or holes. Equally, drying out the plaster and repapering the walls is likely to have a much longer lasting effect if the leaking pipe behind the plaster is sealed up first. That manicure is going to keep his nails looking good much longer if the nail-biting habit is resolved first.

It seemed like Steve understood and agreed with my descriptions, that my analogies made sense to him. I was able to tell him that I believed LCH was likely to be beneficial for him and would be happy to treat him. I gave the normal guidance about the part he would need to play in the process, the CD practice, what to do, how and why to do it.

In my analogy, holes in boats or leaking pipes behind the plaster are the unintentional, accidental, inadvertently misunderstood incidents and events

that the conscious mind has long-forgotten but the subconscious mind is still regarding as a fact or a truth that is indisputable.

To fix those holes, the subconscious mind is invited to work with me to trace the damp back to its source and then it needs to do some remedial work.

The subconscious is the back-room guy who doesn't normally engage with the public but the normal way the conscious and subconscious mind interact with each other and the outside world hasn't yet managed to fix the holes so we need to interact differently.

The CD practice is designed to help the conscious mind gradually get used to going off duty and to help the subconscious mind come forward just far enough for me to communicate with it and join forces with it in this process of finding holes and repairing them.

So would Steve like to go ahead with treatment?

The answer was a definite Yes.

The next step was to show him what hypnosis was going to be like for him. He was a bit unsure about how much he would be aware and was reassured to hear that he would stay in control and could relax as much or as little as felt right to him for that first experience. He put his feet up and I started the induction and he waited for something to happen, decided nothing was going to happen, and then realised that he was actually beginning to relax.

His first words at the end of that time started with "Wow!" He hadn't expected it to affect him that way and was surprised to learn that what had felt about 5 or 10 minutes was actually 25. He'd enjoyed the experience and saw the difference between LCH hypnosis and a deeper trance that he associated with stage hypnosis.

I learnt later that he had thought '*I'd be knocked out cold, like the contestants on a hypnotist's stage show, with no memory of what happened while I was asleep*'. He didn't feel hypnotised, felt like he was in control at all times. He knew he could come out of hypnosis at any time if he wanted to, but he hadn't wanted to. He had been enjoying that unaccustomed depth of relaxation.

We booked the next session. I gave him his CD and the printed reminder of how to practise.

Session 2 – 10 days later

Steve had played the CD nearly every day and had enjoyed it although he had struggled with my previous instructions. This struggle is something that happens to lots of other people, and I totally understand that. I'm continually aiming to improve my explanations, but that's not the whole story.

LCH relies on the client learning a method of responding that is outside of the experience of most people prior to coming for treatment. When something is totally new to us and quite different from what we are accustomed to, we need to hear it a few times before we can really be sure we've heard it correctly and understood it accurately. The response we need from the client during treatment is simple but different, so once people get the hang of it, it's quite easy.

It's an important message to get across that we all respond in our own individual ways, and that's exactly how it's meant to be. A weight lifter is unlikely to be as flexible as a gymnast. An inventor is unlikely to be a meticulous housekeeper. A pregnant woman is unlikely to feel the urge to participate in extreme sports, however much of an adrenaline junkie she was in her younger years.

This is how Steve responded in his own way.

He tried to listen to my words but found himself mentally drifting off. He tried using will-power but was soon too relaxed to prevent himself day-dreaming. He was doing his best to stay with my voice but kept finding himself mentally far, far away. Sometimes he found his imagination has taken him to the memory of the beach where he had enjoyed soaking up the sun and the sea breezes in Tenerife on a recent holiday.

He had some idea of what was required because of my explanations in Session 1 and the CD Notes handout I'd given him, but his logical mind couldn't reconcile the need to listen to the CD and allow himself to mentally drift off at the same time.

We discussed the two parts of the mind, the differences between them and the roles that each of them play.

He agreed that, from time to time, in a room full of people, totally engrossed in a conversation, he would suddenly notice that someone at the other side of the room had said his name. He hadn't previously questioned it, hadn't wondered how that could happen, but started to analyse it now.

In that kind of scenario, he wouldn't have been monitoring the earlier part of that other person's conversation, wouldn't have noticed the remarks leading up to it, but would suddenly have found himself aware of his own name being said and the words that followed it. He began to allow for the possibility that that might have been the result of a constantly vigilant subconscious mind giving him a mental nudge to direct his attention to something relevant to him personally.

In order for us to be aware of what we want and need to know about, and for us not to be overwhelmed with everything else that is going on in our vicinity, the subconscious must be doing some processing and filtering. Like the news team deciding what needs to be included in the headlines, that part of the mind must be shielding us from all the information around us that we don't need to know about.

That little light-bulb moment helped him to take my guidance literally and allow his attention to wander, knowing, with confidence, that the hidden part of his mind was monitoring and would let him know when it was time to come back to his regular level of alertness again. Having sorted out that dilemma, he would be able to practise more easily with his CD following this session.

In the second session, the deeper level of relaxation and the specific guidance included in it resulted in a familiar memory coming into his mind. It was an old family story about something that had happened to him as a child. He didn't know why that memory had come to him then as he hadn't made any logical connection between that event and his nail-biting habit, but he was feeling relaxed and at first, found it easy to go along with it.

In the normal progression of session 2 towards a more detached, less consciously active flow of information, I was aiming to allow for us to move beyond any initial memory, but Steve wasn't able to follow my guidance. He wanted to, but found his attention being held firmly on that early and memorable event.

LCH is based on giving a more prominent voice to that part of the mind that usually plays its part more indirectly and from the background. Steve's conscious mind wasn't driving this in any way. Steve wasn't trying to tell me his theory of what lay at the root of his nail-biting habit. I needed to listen to what Steve had felt a powerful but puzzling and therefore subconsciously driven urge to tell me.

As a typical 5-year old boy, he'd been playing in the garden. He'd been showing off his golf swing. He felt good. He looked good. He was enjoying himself until the club's momentum, at the height of its swing,

slipped out of his fairly strong – for a 5 year old – grip.
It left his hands and flew towards the house. Sod's Law
guided it towards the kitchen window which smashed
and showered the kitchen in broken glass. His younger
brother, then aged about 3 years old, suffered slight
harm. A little bit of blood goes a long way and a little
3 year old can feel very scared and make his feelings
very clear in such a situation.

But I don't think that that was what was at the root of
the nail-biting because it was a well-remembered
incident. It had been dissected, discussed, analysed,
described and enjoyed by all for many years. The young
age of Steve at that time and the lack of intention of
Steve to hurt his brother in any way at that time were
both facts that were quickly acknowledged by all
concerned.

It's very unlikely that that incident had been at the
root of Steve's nail-biting because the subsequent
discussion would have diffused the effects of that
unfortunate accident long before he had reached
adulthood. What he remembered could be part of
the roots, but not the whole of them because it
was out in the clear light of day. It's unlikely that a
misunderstanding of those remembered details could
be hidden from that frequent discussion.

And if it had been at or near the root of Steve's nail-
biting, there would still be some work to do with the
subconscious mind, to find the connection between that
incident and the unwanted habit. We'd need to find
out why that incident had the effect it had, help any

misunderstanding get corrected and help join the
dots between the incident and the symptom. The
subconscious would eventually remove the symptom
once all the erroneous roots had been found and dug up.

But as the information was something Steve felt a
puzzling urge to tell me about, that meant, to me,
that his subconscious mind believed it was relevant
to the development of the nail-biting habit.

It can help to think of the process of LCH treatment as
a retracing of steps back from the present day suffering
of some kind of symptom back along that circuitous
route to the first step of many that brought the client
to need some help. If I need to go by train to London,
then first I need to get to the station. I can't get on the
train from my own front door. There is a leg of that
reversed journey that needs to be completed first.
Session 2 often provides the taxi, the bus or the bracing
walk in the early morning sunshine. It doesn't matter
which route or mode of transport was used. What
matters is that we got to the station on time.

Steve's subconscious seemed to me to be helping
already and needed encouragement to continue doing
that. As for his conscious mind, Steve understood that
I didn't need him to think of any information to give
me. He was willing and able and ready to play his part
in stepping back so his subconscious mind could come
forward to the microphone.

With another appointment booked and clutching a
different CD, knowing exactly how to make the best

use of those practice sessions, Steve left with even better understanding of LCH and a feeling that he was on the right path towards a successful outcome.

Session 3 – 1 week later

He arrived reporting feeling a little bit more chilled than he was accustomed to. Things that would normally have got under his skin were bothering him less since session 2. But we had a challenge to deal with. My normal method of treatment wasn't fitting exactly with Steve's subconscious' eagerness to give me information.

Part of the way we help the conscious mind to distance itself from the information transfer is to use Yes/No questioning. If we ask our clients to describe various aspects of a scene unfolding in their imagination, like the one Steve experienced when the memory of the golf club and the kitchen window came back to him, they need to think and choose the words to best describe it. That requires quite a significant amount of conscious involvement. We progress in Session 3 to closed questions. We simply require a Yes or No which needs no thought or speculation or deliberation.

It generally works really well but early on in Steve's treatment, it had the drawbacks and frustration of being a witness under cross-examination in a court of law. His subconscious seemed to be giving him a specific piece of information to pass on but he was only able to answer the questions I had asked. He had no idea why he was being urged to pass on the specific detail, but knew that, as soon as he heard a certain word, he was to answer 'Yes'. As the questioning continued and that word was never mentioned, Steve found himself experiencing rapid eye movements which were quite uncomfortable.

At the end of that day's treatment, Steve explained and described his experience. We agreed a signal for him to indicate that some verbal information was available, so I could allow it to be delivered and Steve's eyes could relax once again.

Having acknowledged once again that Steve's subconscious mind appeared to be working most constructively with me, giving a clear impression that that part of his mind was keen to help speed the process along, and having agreed a way of opening up that line of communication, Steve's creative and inventive subconscious found a means of working my way, so that signal was never needed, never used in practice.

Session 4 – 1 week later

Even though we hadn't discussed it specifically, Steve had come up with a cracking technique to help him take his attention, his conscious mind, off somewhere else. He had decided to mentally practise a photography presentation while I was asking questions in future sessions. To help himself achieve that, he had already been practising that technique with the CD. The conscious and subconscious parts of his mind were both doing a great job!

As he knew he needed a way for information to come across without his conscious mind getting involved, his creative, imaginative mind, both conscious and subconscious parts together, found a way.

Other clients simply find the Yes or No just comes to them automatically, like the teenager glued to the TV or computer screen giving the appropriate Yes or No to Mum's tea-time interrogation. "Do you want chips with your fish fingers? Yes. Will you start your homework after your tea? Yes. Have you got much homework tonight? No."

Steve seemed to have his own way. No one else that I have treated has ever described such an experience to me. It was totally novel and it seemed to work effectively and efficiently.

Cartoon characters began appearing in his imagination as the questions started flowing. Sometimes an animal or bird was sitting on a ledge or wall and jumping down to the left or right to indicate an answer. The convention he worked with was 'right meant Yes, left meant No'.

At other times, he found himself in a car, and sometimes it was more surreal, in a rocket ship. He was on auto pilot. When each question was asked, he would find the vehicle taking a left or a right turn. He passed that information on while enjoying the imagined journey or the cartoon characters' adventures.

He allowed himself to get thoroughly engrossed in the scenes unfolding before him, which had no relevance to the questions I was asking. They simply provided the answers. He was oblivious to my questions.

The only way I could make sense of that experience was that his subconscious was engineering these images to give me information. It's similar to the way a sound like the alarm clock or a knocking at the door get woven into a dream as the phone ringing or someone hammering a nail in. As we wake, the true meaning of the sounds becomes clear as the dream fades.

The answers came through for each and every question and seemed to be making enough sense to me so that I was able to work constructively with the information I was receiving.

The images changed throughout treatment and Steve was happy to be passive in that process. He wanted his subconscious to provide me with the information because he clearly understood that that was the key to successful and efficient treatment, to the speedy arrival at the desired outcome. He found it easy to distance himself from the questions themselves by simply watching the cartoons unfold in front of him and get entertained by that instead.

His subconscious was holding the TV remote control and he, his conscious mind, was being given coded information to pass on to me in the process.

That happened nearly all the way through, except at one point in the questioning. It seemed like, however hard he tried, his subconscious mind wouldn't let him drift away from the questions. He felt as if his attention was being demanded. He soon found it was useless to resist so he paid attention briefly. He then found himself being allowed to drift off back to the cartoon again.

We discussed this afterwards and I suggested it might have been like in a business situation, in a partnership. Each partner specialises in their own field of the business, happy to let the other get on with their core role. From time to time, something more crucial is being considered. The decision is too big for one of them to decide on their own. Maybe the whole business would be at stake. Maybe it related to a contract too big to be allowed to be taken on or rejected single-handedly so, briefly, they get together and get up to speed on all the relevant information. They would need to check that all key issues had been considered and then make a joint decision, to sign or not as appropriate. Then they'd get back to specialising on their own normal separate roles for efficiency.

Steve agreed that that's what it felt like. He didn't know what it was about, but he knew it was important. He hadn't actually been consciously involved but it was as if he needed to be in the room, available if needed at any point. He had got the rapid eye movement and feelings of frustration again during that period of conscious involvement, just like in the previous session.

And as questioning continued, sometimes it would be a cat and a canary, either the much-loved pets at home or the classic Warner Bros Sylvester and Tweety. Pause for the inevitable, in the interests of accuracy – got to get the spelling wight. I just had to watch several clips... I taught I taw a puddy cat on YouTube – and managed to... ahem... drag myself back within an hour or so to my current task, making a mental note to go back and enjoy more once the first draft of the next chapter is complete.

Sometimes, a huge cartoon hammer would hit his right or left hand and he'd pass on the appropriate yes or no while continuing to follow the adventures of that wily feline and the appealing yellow cutey all kept in their places by the firm but fair greying granny. I know how he felt. It's so easy to get engrossed. I'd better close down that internet session before another childhood Looney Tunes memory tugs at my attention.

Towards the end of that session, he had a different kind of experience. It had a dream-like quality to it, and again, no other client has described anything quite like it. It didn't have any connection with anything I'd said to him either in discussion or under hypnosis. It seemed like his nail-biting habit had turned into some item of rubbish that was being dropped into a cartoon dustbin. Then a giant cartoon boot kicked it away into the distance in a cloud of dust.

At end of the hypnosis, while I was counting down from 7 to 1 to gently bring him back to wide awake, he saw another of those strange images play out in front of him, although his eyes were still closed at the time. He watched with fascination as his hands appeared in front of his face with his fingers and nails facing towards him. Each count was matched or mirrored by a jerky movement of his hands another inch or so further away from his face. At the count of 1, the hands were replaced by a bright light, a feeling of 'wow!' a sense of relief or release, like an emotional lifting of a great weight. He felt like he was saying goodbye to something.

He felt different as he walked out of the room that day.

Some people have described a sense of happiness or relief or even momentary sadness or regret, without having any idea why. They were happily day-dreaming at the time, so it was a totally puzzling experience to them. One lady was convinced that a tear had rolled down her cheek but there was no thought or feeling attached to it. She didn't have any memory come to her at the time and felt emotionally calm and relaxed. She could clearly feel its wetness travel down from the corner of her eye, but after the hypnosis, there was no sign of there having actually been a tear.

So it's not that rare to have puzzling experiences, but Steve's were in glorious technicolour and at times, spookily relevant to what we could theorise was going on in treatment.

He had clearly had a eureka moment but I wasn't expecting that to be it. It's quite unusual for there to be just one key incident, and to find it on the first full session of questioning, so we booked a session for the following week. Steve had an instinct that that session had been significant, but went along with my advice without commenting.

During the week, he got in touch to rearrange the session. He was very busy that week and things were going really well with his nail-biting. It was already beginning to reduce in frequency and intensity. He was beginning to notice his fingers moving towards his mouth so he could decide to stop them in their tracks. It still took a bit of effort, but it was getting easier.

We rebooked for about 4 weeks on from that session, which is an average amount of time to allow for further processing. The subconscious is doing the equivalent, in that time, of totting up a huge column of figures. It needs time to complete that task and reach a total before we ask any further questions.

Session 5 – 4 weeks later

Steve was proud to show me his totally un-bitten nails, now neatly manicured. Any broken skin or damaged nail he'd noticed was now a prompt to go fetch a pair of scissors to tidy it up properly. The session consisted of a thorough check of all subconscious information that had led to the symptom. The cartoon characters continued to provide the information while keeping Steve amused and entertained with the comical animal adventures. With the information available at that time, there were no remaining stray roots needing attention and his subconscious confirmed that there was no further need for Steve to bite his nails.

There didn't seem to be any signs for concern but
I explained that I can't guarantee happily ever after.
I related it to tidying up a garage or shed, an attic or
cellar full of boxes, bin-liners, old suitcases. Once most
have been checked and found to contain only rubbish,
they can be easily cleared out. If his nail-biting were
to creep back in at any point, I wouldn't want him to
draw the conclusion that it hadn't worked, that it had
been a short-term fix, like the other measures he'd
tried. I'd prefer to leave him knowing that it was more
likely to be a tiny box or bag that had been lurking in a
corner and had contained another incident that needed
examining and reassessing. Another session or two
would be likely to be all that was required.

So I reinforced that I wasn't expecting his habit to
begin to return, or for it to become an effort to resist
biting again, but if it did, not to be concerned but
instead to simply book another session. He was happy
and relieved to hear that.

CHAPTER 11

Something that seems small at first has the potential to send ripples a long way

And I'm pleased to report that all is still fine since the treatment concluded.

Steve didn't, and still doesn't, want to know the underlying information. He's just happy it's all in the past now. He wants to help others get similar benefits. He's been telling people himself and has given his permission for his story to be told here. He was highly motivated for his treatment to be a success, for himself, but also for me!

It's no longer on his mind, that annoying and unwelcome habit that had, for many years, added another layer of irritation and concern to the normal stresses and challenges of running a business.

That one fly in the ointment has now gone and he is busy getting on with what he does so well.

His words seem to sum it up nicely. "How the heck did that happen?"

Pat wanted to know the answers to a few extra questions I hadn't included in my notes. I've copied Steve's replies without amending or paraphrasing, as I think it's so valuable to be able to report exactly what my clients say, in their own words, about their treatment.

Pat: *Why did you choose or consider hypnotherapy?*

Steve: *It was a last resort. Willpower and pharmacy products had all failed. For some reason, I knew hypnotherapy would work, but I didn't know why*

Pat: *What did you understand of hypnotherapy and LCH before deciding to book in for treatment?*

Steve: *Absolutely nothing. I think it's an industry that nobody knows anything about, apart from the people involved in it. Like most people I thought I'd be knocked out cold, like the contestants on a hypnotist's stage show, with no memory of what happened while I was asleep.*

Pat: *What had that conversation at the networking meeting told you?*

Steve: *That treatment was totally different. I thought I would be hypnotised and then repeatedly told 'not to bite my nails' but it doesn't work like that. Treatment involves finding the reason why I'm biting my nails, which takes a careful process.*

Pat: *What impression had that meeting left you with?*

Steve: *Just do it – have the treatment, and after meeting Mary I had faith and trust in her that she could solve the problem.*

Pat: *And how are you getting on now? Did the
       habit return? Did you need any more sessions?*

Steve: *I haven't bitten my nails since...even once!
       I sometimes put my fingers in my mouth and
       tap my teeth with my nails, but I've never
       bitten them. It's a weird feeling that I can't
       explain. I have no inclination or desire to
       bite them at all. It's like I never have. I'm
       proud of my hands. In fact I joke now that
       I'm fed up cutting my nails all the time with
       nail-clippers!!*

Me: Pat and Chris – what are the main messages
       from this case?

Pat: *I've been thinking about what kinds of
       symptoms are worth spending money on to
       pay for treatment. Nail-biting doesn't sound
       like something that serious. I don't think
       I would have considered going to see a
       therapist.*

Chris: *That's what I started out thinking, but then
       I remembered what Steve said about his
       business. He needs to pitch to prospective
       clients. First impressions are important and the
       most powerful forces often come from things we
       don't actually notice and think about. We just let
       our instincts guide us. A contract could have
       been lost because Steve's nails led to an overall
       impression that something wasn't quite right.
       That contract could have made a difference to
       his business as a whole, the wellbeing of his
       family and the jobs of his employees.*

Pat: *Well if that's true, then the cost of treatment is relatively minor in comparison. And I guess that, even if he never lost a contract that way, if he was often worrying that he might, then the peace of mind he has now is well worth the money he spent. Something that seems quite small when you first look at it has the potential to send ripples out a long way.*

CHAPTER 12

What would it take for us to
even consider the possibility?

**Pat and Chris are interested in knowing more about
treating a physical symptom**

Chris: *In 'What if...' you described the treatment you
had for your own physical symptom. What first
made you think that LCH was capable of being
effective with something physical?*

    Me: It took me a long time to get my thoughts
together. It was a gradual process of analysing
what I'd observed and heard and read about
from the perspective of various assumptions
about the subconscious mind.

In our traditional Western medicine, research seems to
go steadily in the direction of smaller and smaller, the
cell, the atom, the nucleus, the gene, the DNA. I've
heard that likened to trying to understand the works
of Shakespeare by counting the number of words or
letters, by analysing how many a's and b's and c's.

Sometimes we can get so focussed on greater detail,
especially as microscopes and other scientific instruments

become more and more sensitive, that we can miss out on all the other information we would get if we stepped back to see the whole picture in one go.

I stepped back and looked at the subconscious mind as if it were a person. I reasoned that there are so many different kinds of people that it's highly likely that I can think of one that describes what the subconscious is doing at any particular time, and much more importantly, why.

I don't really concern myself too much with 'how'. I don't have those scientific skills. Like the police in a major crime investigation, one key factor for me is 'motive' and another key factor is never to underestimate the power of the subconscious. I don't need to know 'how' a physical effect is created. I just believe, and have witnessed it work, and create changes which can seem miraculous at times. This is enough for me until we understand more about the process.

People often say "I'll believe it when I see it", but maybe the truth is more that "I'll see it when I believe it". I certainly want to believe it, partly because it seems to open up some new possibilities for our health, and partly because it seems to make sense of some otherwise puzzling observations.

Setting the scene for treating physical health conditions in the context of my career to date

I'd done the LCH Home Study in 2005 and the Practical Course in spring 2006. I had completed

5 of the 9 Diploma Modules and was working on Module 6. I'd been in practice part time from the summer of 2006 to the end of 2007, at which point, I took voluntary redundancy from my programming job of 20+ years and began to put all my working time and effort into LCH.

People came to me for help with addictions and phobias, insomnia and anxiety, panic attacks, low self esteem, to stop smoking and lose weight. These, and similar conditions and issues are the kind for which people often consider hypnotherapy as being an appropriate and promising form of therapy or intervention.

I hadn't, up to that point, treated anyone with a physical symptom. It's not really surprising because not many people would consider hypnotherapy for something physical. Most people wouldn't do an internet search for hypnotherapists in their area if they had a physical symptom unless they had reason to believe or at least suspect a psychological connection.

But if I only ever get a skin rash or breathing difficulties when the exam season is looming, then as soon as I spot that pattern emerging, I might just consider that it isn't purely physical.

The phone and the gas fitters

My phone stopped working. I rang the phone company. The engineer came to my house and did some investigations, followed clues and cables, used diagnostic equipment, moved furniture, lifted floorboards, and eventually found the cause. He discovered a section of cable that had been damaged by heat, a lot of heat.

A little while previously, I can't remember exactly how long before, I'd had some work done on my central heating system. They had replaced an old fire-back boiler with a new and more energy efficient one that was relocated into what had previously been the airing cupboard. Lots of the pipe work had to be re-routed in the process.

Presumably, the gas engineer hadn't noticed that he was heating up some telephone cables at the time of all that work on the pipes. The first time I tried to use the land line after the gas engineer had inadvertently melted the phone cable, the dialling tone was missing. Like most people nowadays, I have various phones, and use some more than others, so there could have been a few days elapsed before I noticed the phone fault.

Even if the two events had been back to back, I don't know what would have made me suspect a connection between them. I had a boiler fitted. My land-line stopped working. That is surely just an example of two totally unconnected events that just happened to take place one after the other.

The telephone engineer replaced the section of welded cable with a new section and the phone sprang back into life. Then he gave me the bad news. As the fault wasn't theirs, the telephone company would be sending me a bill of £100 for their engineer's time. As we had already worked out by then that it must have been caused by the gas engineer's work, he suggested I pay the bill and then claim the money back from the company that fitted the boiler. He left me the appropriate paperwork, with his findings documented, and also the burnt section of cable.

When I contacted the boiler fitters, they sent someone round to assess my claim. The investigator was prepared to agree that his engineer had done the damage that had resulted in my phone not working. He didn't want to pay the £100, though, and complained that I should have rung him up in the first place, thus saving the £100. I'm not sure how he thought a gas engineer would have been able to locate and fix the faulty section of phone cable without the appropriate skills and the telephone diagnostic equipment.

I was even more puzzled as to how he expected me to infer from the failure in the phone line that the best course of action would be to contact the gas engineer! I would have got a very puzzled reply from the person I got through to on the boiler company's customer service number if I explained that I was calling them for assistance as my phone wasn't working.

That was a long story used to illustrate that we might never think of hypnotherapy to fix a physical symptom any more than we might think that a gas engineer had caused a fault on a land line – unless, like me, we had some previous experience to cause us to consider the possibility.

When you know the extra information, with the wonderful gift of hindsight, it's quite a logical progression of events, not bizarre in any way. Without the extra information, what would it take for us to even consider the possibility?

The mind and the body – the link between then

All the way through my training, I had learnt more and more about the subconscious mind. I had begun to view it as something like the centre of command of the Starship Enterprise. Everything that needed to be initiated, balanced, co-ordinated, monitored and adjusted would need input from that command centre.

Blushing and fainting are two simple examples of physical changes that can take place as a result of activity in the mind.

For example, I said something that had a double meaning, the second meaning of which I'd not intended and wasn't one I would have chosen to air in present company. As soon as those words left my lips, that other meaning hit me!

I felt embarrassed and people could see that because my face reddened, which might actually make me feel even worse, even more embarrassed. That reddening, that blushing, isn't something I can make happen using willpower. It involves certain blood vessels dilating and extra blood getting diverted to the face and neck. There is no conscious control mechanism for that blood movement.

Some people faint at the sight of blood. We can faint
for all sorts of reasons that are quite simply physical,
such as giving blood when we haven't eaten enough in
the previous few hours. Fainting at the sight of blood,
someone else's blood, that doesn't have a physical
cause like dehydration or low blood sugar. Fainting,
like blushing, is the result of an abnormal situation in
the flow of blood.

If our blood pressure drops suddenly and severely, then
certain vital organs can be at risk of being deprived of
nutrients which could cause severe and permanent
damage. The body has its own correction mechanism
in place which helps minimise the risk to the most vital
organ, the brain itself. It causes a loss of consciousness
and a fall to the floor, where, in that position, more
of the blood will be able to reach the brain because it
doesn't have to fight against gravity.

For that mechanism to kick in for no other reason than
the sight of someone else's blood, then it can't be a
purely physical mechanism. There must be a form of
intelligence that is receiving the information from the
eyes, combining it with information stored in the brain's
database, creating an interpretation, adding some
meaning to the information gained and eventually
determining the best course of action. If there's a need
to get out of the situation, for some reason, then the
physical reaction results in that need being met.
The person is 'out of it' for the duration of the faint.

Some significant source of intelligence had to be
available for all of that sensing, processing, analysing,

and reacting to have taken place, and other than the
original awareness of the sight of the blood, no part
of it was conscious. We can't make ourselves faint at
will, and it's hard to imagine a reason why anyone
would want that outcome. It's quite an unpleasant
experience and one we would try to avoid once we'd
been there and were able to recognise the signs of an
imminent faint.

> **If we simply define the subconscious as the part of
> the mind that's in control of everything that's going
> on within us, everything that is life-supporting but
> also, in contrast, anything that we haven't chosen,
> don't want and can't dispose of, then it's clear to see
> that it's capable of far more than we might, on first
> thought, give it credit for.**

By having that simple definition in mind, I've been able
to look at much of what happens within us from a
totally different angle from the way it looked to me
before I started my training. Fact is so often stranger
than fiction, until we know the rest of the relevant
information, like the gas fitter causing my landline fault.

My training led me to consider that LCH might be able
to improve or even eliminate physical symptoms and
I learnt that other therapists have apparently achieved
those kind of puzzling improvements.

I needed to prove it to myself, prove that I could also
help provide those kinds of benefits, before I could
offer it to my clients. I started by discussing it with
someone I knew had a physical symptom. I didn't even

know how to broach the subject as people can view such a question as insulting and demeaning. I asked a few questions and let the responses guide me as to how far I could take this line of enquiry before backing away and hoping I'd done no harm.

In my wildest dreams, I couldn't have predicted where those first few tentative questions would eventually lead. Pat's curiosity has recently been focussed on the same subject.

Pat: *I've been thinking more and more about LCH. It seems so different from anything else I've looked at. I've heard that anything alternative or complementary is often dismissed as placebo or spontaneous remission by much of the medical and scientific community.*

Are you saying that physical symptoms can be disposed of when LCH treatment is successful?

Me: Yes, I believe they can be and I believe they have been.

Pat: *Apart from your own treatment, the treatment you received, have you any more details you can give? Can you describe anything about treatments you've given and the results you've achieved?*

Me: Yes, I can now. One of my ex-clients, knowing that I was writing a book about the type of treatment he had received from me, offered his permission for me to include some details. All that I'm about to tell you has been approved by him. Although, obviously, I have changed his name, there is enough information here to identify it to some people as probably being his story because he has told lots of people about it.

People close to him, people he has confided in, will probably recognise the details. He has told the story to numerous friends and acquaintances and is happy for people to know of his experience if it will help others benefit from LCH.

Pat: *Ok then, tell me all about it.*

Me: He'd been interested in the new career I'd embarked on right from the start, wanting to know what it was about and how I was getting on. After I'd been in practice part-time for just over a year, I decided that I'd run some ideas by him. I've always been wary about approaching the subject with anyone who has a physical symptom.

> **I recognise that people could see my ideas as implying that their condition is psychosomatic – as 'all in the mind'. Some might then go on to assume I mean that it's not real, or that they could sort it out for themselves if they wanted to and tried hard enough – and I definitely don't believe any of those inferences.**

I expect that many people would feel insulted, would be angry with me, if I made any kind of inference that their physical symptom might have a psychological cause – even if I emphasised that I was referring to the subconscious mind.

I started the discussion on very general terms to see how he responded.

I found out later that he had been very sceptical at first, but had diplomatically kept those thoughts to himself.

Pat: *Tell me more about his scepticism.*

Me: I can do better than that. I have a note he sent me and I'll read it to you word for word.

> *My initial perceptions were based on previous views of hypnotherapy – people being made to act like a dog or some other silly thing on stage. I used to believe hypnotherapy was a bit of a con or at most that the people messing about with it were a bit weird / a bit of a crackpot!*
>
> *Although I knew Mary and nothing that I already knew about her made me think she was a crackpot my initial thought was that I didn't think she was into anything like that and I thought that she had a secret life other than the one I knew.*
>
> *However, all that I did know about Mary was at odds with the thought she would want to be on a stage (she was very quiet and reserved) or more particularly that she would want to humiliate anyone. This gave me some pause for thought,*

however, I cannot claim that it was mostly those reasons that made me listen more to Mary. I think that mostly I was just making conversation and she was obviously passionate about it.

As her concern for other people's well being came through I began to be genuinely interested in what she had to say about what she did. Also as Mary was a very reserved person and I could tell when she came to speak to me about treating me that she was obviously out of her own comfort zone coming to speak to me about it I thought it must be important.

Whenever I talk to anyone about my own experience I can see them switch off to what I say (in much the same way as if I talk about my engineering job) and I see them start to think I'm a bit crazy/weird/ fruit loop...

I also thought that I would be 'put under'/ brainwash me or not be aware of what was happening. This never occurred. I was always aware of what was happening and Mary never tried to 'trick me' into believing anything differently. All she ever seemed to do was to trace back a series of events (some of which 'popped' into my mind as she asked about them) and ask me whether I now agreed with the conclusions I had drawn from the event.

These are some of the kinds of ideas we discussed.
If something doesn't have an external cause, it must
have an internal cause. Even if it has an external cause,
there's rarely an illness or disease that affects everyone
equally. When there's a virus or bacterial infection
going around, some suffer more than others, and some
escape it totally. We could imagine there being some
kind of control centre, something that tells the brain to
send those signals to the organs and systems within the
body that do things like fight infections, mend broken
bones, cause minor cuts and grazes to scab over.

We could question whether there is something causing
some people to only get colds at the weekend or when
they're on holiday and others to be ill only when they
are in the middle of an important work project.

I hadn't treated anyone for a physical symptom before
but knew that my colleagues had had success with
various physical conditions. I couldn't offer any kind
of confidence at that point, so asked if he would be
prepared to give it a try – no fee. It would be for
mutual benefit as I would be able to treat other people
with more confidence – and if it failed, or took a lot of
sessions, it would cost him some time but no money.

He has a scientific background – a PhD in something
far outside my ability to take in more than the simplest
of explanations so I was surprised and impressed that
he was so ready to take on my every-day kinds of ideas
and explanations. He was keen to give it a try.

CHAPTER 13

Thought you might like 2 know that yesterday I had a chip butty and a beer and I'm still ok!

Pat: *We've been through all that theoretical information and it makes sense to me that the subconscious is in control of far more than we might first think. You've treated at least one person for a physical symptom, and that person is happy for you to tell his story, so take us through it so we can see for ourselves.*

Me: Ok. He would be ill if he ate the tiniest amount of gluten.

Pat: *Ill in what way?*

Me: Severe diarrhoea continuing until all traces of the gluten had been got rid of from the digestive system. He gave one example of how tiny was the amount that would affect him. He couldn't eat chips from the fish and chip shop.

Chris: *Hang on. There's no gluten in chips. They're just potato and oil. Why did that make him ill?*

Me: Many chip-shops cook the fish and the chips in the same oil. The fish is coated in batter made with flour that contains gluten and even if it was small enough to be invisible, it was there in sufficient quantity to make him ill. Even if they cook fish and chips in separate fryers, the staff constantly handle both, so cross-contamination is inevitable.

Chris: *Ok – that's quite severe. But if a talking therapy such as LCH took it away, then might it have been all in his mind in the first place? Maybe he was just ill because he thought he'd eaten gluten. Maybe the first time he was ill, the food was contaminated in some way, maybe it had gone off, but he believed it was gluten that caused his illness.*

Me: He had various restaurants and takeaways whose food he could safely eat. From time to time, however careful he was about his diet, he would find himself ill again. Usually, he would eventually track it down and find that where or what he had just eaten, they'd changed the recipe and it was no longer gluten-free.

Secondly, does it matter whether it's all in the mind?

Chris: *It might matter to the sufferer. They might judge themselves, feel it was their fault. They might consider that they should be able to 'pull themselves together' because it isn't a 'real' illness. Even if they don't judge themselves, others might see it that way and criticise them for it.*

Me: The sufferer didn't choose to be so ill, doesn't want the reaction of their body to be so extreme for a food ingredient that is present in so much of today's processed food. Home cooked food containing certain types of flours and grains also act like a poison for many people. Would it be fair for anyone, the sufferer or anyone else, to judge the sufferer for something that causes such unpleasant symptoms?

Chris: *No, it isn't fair but it happens and it hurts.*

Me: I agree, and that's another reason to work towards resolving it.

Do you know what the medical treatment is for gluten intolerance?

Pat: *I don't think it's regarded as curable. They are just advised to keep their diet totally gluten-free. That's getting easier as even supermarkets have a wide range of gluten-free food that is getting closer in taste and in price to the standard equivalents.*

Me: So what would be the 'magic wand' outcome in this case?

Chris: *They found a cure. The pharmaceutical companies developed medication that cures the condition.*

Pat: *Yes, it would be a small price to pay to take a pill, once a day, or even several times a day, if they could then eat what they wanted. Or maybe an operation that corrected whatever it was in the stomach that is different in those with the intolerance. It's something about the villi, I think.*

I read something on the NHS website and it seemed to be saying that it's an autoimmune response. What you said about it acting like a poison seems to fit with what they described. It's as if the body detects the gluten and decides that it's a threat to the body. It creates an inflammation to fight the threat. The inflammation prevents the 'poison' from being absorbed but it achieves that in a drastic way. It prevents all the food from being absorbed, including the healthy ingredients.

The villi are part of the way the stomach absorbs nutrients. They are finger-shaped structures in the stomach lining that greatly increase the surface area that the food can be absorbed through. The inflammation stops them from doing their job properly. The villi flatten and join together. Maybe they are forming a shield against the perceived malicious intruder.

If someone with this condition continues to eat gluten, they'll begin to suffer from malnutrition. Before it was discovered that gluten was the culprit and the safe diet was found, people became extremely ill and eventually died from it.

Me: That's what I've interpreted too. It seems that the intolerance is often diagnosed as Coeliac disease. Coeliac.org.uk describes the villi getting damaged, flattened together and in severe cases, completely disappearing. If people have only mild symptoms and continue to eat gluten because they don't know why they feel under the weather, tired and listless, lacking in motivation, then the result can be mild osteoporosis and anaemia. The body isn't absorbing enough of the calcium and iron from their food to keep them fit and well.

Pat: *Was the person who came to you diagnosed with Coeliac disease?*

Me: Yes, he was diagnosed and given a prescription for free gluten-free food. He was given that diagnosis because his symptoms were identical to the classic Coeliac pattern – eat gluten, be very ill, don't eat gluten, stay totally well and healthy.

Chris: *So we wave a magic wand and they find a cure and he has life-changing surgery or he takes a pill that keeps it under control, and either way, he can eat what he wants and doesn't suffer those symptoms any more.*

Pat: *But you're not a surgeon or a GP or a medical scientist, so what did you do?*

Me: What would you think of those benefits without the surgery, without the pills?

Pat: *I don't want to seem dismissive, but how can you and LCH achieve something that the NHS hasn't managed? I've known you for years and you're not a genius, so is LCH magic?*

Me: I'd really like someone to do some research
      and establish what went on for some of the
      people that LCH has helped so that it can
      be more broadly used where it would be
      beneficial. The man with the adverse reaction
      to gluten feels the same.

Pat: *Ok, we're sitting comfortably...*

What led to treatment

I knew that Bill was a scientist, and that he was
interested in learning about the hypnotherapy training
I'd had and what results I'd achieved. I asked him if he
would be interested in discussing his gluten intolerance
with reference to LCH, purely to help me learn how to
broach that delicate subject.

I wanted to be able to tell people that there was a
possibility that a medical 'end of the line' wasn't
necessarily a life-sentence. In situations where no
diagnosis could be made, or a diagnosis was made
but the recommended treatment was unsuccessful, or,
as in his case, the recommended course of action was
avoidance of the trigger food or situation or whatever
sparked off the symptoms, there is still another avenue
to pursue.

He wanted to be able to eat in a cafe or restaurant or
from a shop or takeaway without having to read labels
carefully or ask loads of questions and still worry in
case there was some tiny amount of gluten in what he
was eating.

He wanted to be able to eat without worrying about getting ill – very ill.

He wanted to be able to eat with other people, accept other people's hospitality, share food at other people's parties.

There is a medical test for this disease, but in order for the test to be carried out, the sufferer has to eat an unrestricted diet containing gluten for 6 to 8 weeks, which would have been horrendous for him. It would have been so very painful and would have so severely disrupted his life, possibly even kept him house-bound for a couple of months, and could have left him weak and malnourished and needing many more weeks to recuperate and return to his previous normal state of health.

Bill had been told that, whether he went for the Coeliac test or not, and if he did, whether or not it was conclusive, the treatment was the same - nothing. The only advice would be to avoid even the tiniest amount of gluten. It was a diet-controlled condition. His doctor wanted to have the certainty of the test result, but couldn't recommend such a drastic experience for Bill because there would be no reward, no benefit at all in establishing the outcome of the test.

We discussed, in very general terms, when a thought or a feeling cause a physical change. If someone isn't born with a condition, then something must have triggered it off. Something must have loaded the gun in the first place because an empty gun just makes a click and doesn't do any harm or damage. If the cause isn't external, then we can argue that means that it's necessarily internal.

Bill asked if I was suggesting treating him and went away to think it over. I went away and all my concerns came rushing in. I feared a negative response to the discussion itself.

He had taken intense interest, had listened and considered all I'd said, had discussed it with his wife and wanted me to treat him. He had long been craving toast and scones and biscuits that most of us take for granted. He really wanted to be able to grab a sandwich or a pasty or a pie when hungry. Keeping his stock of meals and nibbles topped up with tasty food he could safely eat took a lot of time home-baking and a lot of money. The gluten-free ingredients were always more expensive than the standard variety.

I explained to him that I had no way of knowing if there was any chance of success, so would not want to charge any kind of fee – that I would greatly appreciate his time and cooperation on the basis that it would have the potential to be beneficial to both of us. Also, other than taking his time and mine, I knew of no other possible risk or negative side-effects.

We agreed to start treatment mid January 2008. I had been as honest as I could about the fact that I had no personal track record on physical symptoms and was not charging any money.

We both wanted to believe it. We both wanted to see it.

Bill remembers the discussion we had

My memory of the conversation was quite vague. It happened in late 2007. I needed his help and he emailed me his memory of how it went.

Me: Why do you have this allergy?

Bill: *Because my body reacts to gluten*

Me: Why?

Bill: *because gluten causes the villi in my intestines to flatten which leads to malnourishment*

(http://celiacdisease.about.com/od/symptoms ofceliacdisease/a/celiacsymptoms.htm)

Me: Why does your body do that?

Bill: *I don't know, it just does*

Me: Has it always done it?

Bill: *No*

Me: Does it happen to everyone who eats gluten?

Bill: *No*

Me: Then why you?

Bill: *I don't know.*

Me: Why has it started now?

Bill: *I don't know*

Me: Could it be something internal that has caused this to start? If it was an external cause then other people who have the same food and live in the same environments should have the same symptoms.

Bill: *How could that happen, is there something wrong with me?*

Me: No but we all have a subconscious part of our minds that works like a computer. Based on using very simple logic. That part of your mind can control things like your symptoms.

Bill: *But if it was working for my good then why would it create something so horrible?*

Me: Sometimes it gets it wrong. For example imagine if you never learnt that Father Christmas wasn't real. You would look at the world in a different way. Or imagine a girl in bed. She hears her mum telling her friend that she cannot come out to play because she is not too bright. She does not know the alternative meaning of the phrase and thinks that her mother thinks that she is not very clever. This may be reinforced through several other events.

This changes the way that she feels about and sees the world and unless she un-learns this then it could lead through many series of other incidents to creating a symptom to avoid herself looking stupid. For example she may develop migraines as an excuse for her to not have to go to a pub quiz or another event where she may look silly. It is never that simple but you can get the idea. What I do is try and trace back the path of events that caused your subconscious to think in this way.

Bill: *But why has my mind not done this already?*
I don't want to be like this.

Me: If you knew where the cause of this was
coming from then in hindsight with your
extra experience then you would already have
solved this yourself. Sometimes your mind
needs a little help to trace back the events. The
hypnotherapy I do just asks your mind why are
you doing this? Your subconscious can then say
because of this reason, from this event and so
on until we reach an original event.

Once your subconscious relooks at the
conclusions it drew from this event it can
correct where it went wrong.

Then it can work back through all the other
conclusions it drew from all the other events
based on the thinking from the first event
which now appears to be wrong. Like a tree
branching out or a root changing direction and
growing distorted because it has hit a stone.
The original event will be something that you
will hardly remember as if you knew about it
you would have solved your problem yourself
already.

Bill: *The other thing I remember talking to you*
about was why LCH was different from other
types of hypnotherapy. Mainly LCH looks at
*the cause. **It also does not ask your mind to***
change or do anything. Your mind does that on
***its own.** LCH just helps it find the original*
event and trace the path. Other types of

hypnotherapy treat the symptoms which if LCH theory is correct will cause a different symptom to fulfil what the subconscious is trying to achieve by creating the symptom in the first place.

I am not an expert in this and this is just my speculation but I believe that the advantages of the symptom were;

Made people feel sorry for me and got them to look after me

Gave me extra attention

Made me "special"

This filled a desire that I was not even properly aware of. After treatment the hard part has been realising this and growing up to fulfil myself in a more productive way. I am not sure if this is too personal for what you want to say in the book but feel free to use it if you want to.

Anyway I have babbled on enough now and I am no expert in LCH so I may have even got the ideas completely wrong! Use whatever you would like to from the above. I am just so grateful for you fixing me that I am willing to help in any way I can and I would love to see others benefit from it too.

His wife added some comments of her own.

I think I was there for some of this conversation. I remember you just kept asking "Why?" I really wanted to find an answer to your questions, but every time we did, you asked "why?" again until we ran out. I didn't want to agree with your opinion, but I couldn't disagree with your logic...

She recently told me that there were three key points that convinced her that this was a promising avenue to try. One was the 'grit in your shoe' analogy described in Chapter 7 of my book 'What if it really is... ?' Another was the story of the little girl hearing her mother describe her as 'not too bright' an expression meaning 'a bit poorly' and taking her mother's words literally – an example she could believe in and understand. The remaining one was the fact that they couldn't answer my repeated queries - 'yes but why?' Why this? Why you? Why now?

Bill's treatment started

It was early in 2008 and we started with the consultation. Gluten made him ill. It caused his body to eject the entire contents of his digestive system within minutes or hours of eating something containing even tiny quantities of gluten.

He was fine, totally symptom-free, if he ate a gluten-free diet. He couldn't eat wheat, oats, barley, rye and spelt, although in the early stages, he'd been able to eat oats.

This kind of worsening suggests to me that there could be some kind of underlying cause that is only indirectly related to the symptom. I've spoken to, read about and heard of, people with intolerances or allergies to certain types of food. Once they identify the offending food, they eliminate it totally from their diet. Things are fine for a while. Then the symptoms return and they continue to suffer until a further rogue food is identified.

Maybe there's a deeply held (subconscious) need to be ill. When that food is found and then totally avoided, then the illness is removed, but not the need to be ill. If someone successfully eliminates specific foods from their diet, then the subconscious would need to create another 'illness'. The simplest solution would be to create a similar adverse reaction to another food type.

As long as that underlying 'need to be ill' remains uncorrected, then each identified and eliminated food type would cause that cycle of illness, identify cause, eliminate cause, well for a while, new food reaction created.

The long-term outcome could be a spiral down into chronic malnutrition. We need to find and dig up the roots so that there's no longer that deep but hidden need to be ill.

Bill was happy to let me guide him on how I needed him to respond so that I could set up a line of communication with his subconscious mind and encourage his conscious mind to steadily reduce its influence on the proceedings.

Early on in treatment, he had asked how he would know when it was ok to eat gluten. I said that he would probably get some kind of feeling, some instinct that would tell him that it was ok. And at that point, he would need to make very small changes to his diet as he continued to follow his instincts.

As we progressed through his treatment, I gained some information which gave me the opportunity to point out to his subconscious mind possible areas for review, re-examination, re-interpretation. The offered suggestions for review seemed to have been taken up. A few days after one session, I got a message from him that showed there were signs of possible improvement.

He had eaten some food that normally contained minute quantities of gluten, food that normally made him ill. He had just known that it was ok to do so. He had felt sure that something significant had happened in that session and that feeling had been followed by an urge to eat something specific. He knew he would be ok – and he was!

He'd eaten it because he'd 'known' it was ok to eat it. He 'knew' he wouldn't be ill. He didn't know how or why he knew that. Putting that into context, he's a scientist who normally relies on facts, information, logic, results or outcomes from concrete, physical interventions - but he let his instincts guide him on that occasion.

Maybe all the discussions we'd had had led him to consider his subconscious in a different way now. Maybe he'd never given that part of his mind a second thought before, but maybe, he'd started to attribute lots of good things in his life to the actions of his conscientious silent virtual partner, to his diligent life-support system.

Memories of incidents

Bill remembered a number of incidents around his primary school teacher. She was everyone's favourite teacher and, in many ways, very good at her job. She put a lot of time and effort, resources and creativity into making her lessons enjoyable as well as inspiring and educational.

But in her dealings with him, there was a completely different atmosphere. In one incident, he'd put his lunch box away before he should have, although he didn't know that at the time. He'd done it before the other children had, and got shouted at by this teacher who demanded to know if he thought he was special.

His mother was a teacher at the same school and she, herself, was being treated badly by the 'favourite' teacher. On reflection, it looks now like the 'favourite' teacher was taking her dislike of his mother out on him.

She shouted at him and then acted as if nothing had happened, which left him with a mixture of feelings that, at that young age, and out on a limb from all his class-mates, were very hard to deal with.

Any child whose mother or father is a teacher at the same school can find themselves in that ambivalent situation of being seen as 'special' in a most unwelcome way.

He was only about 7 or 8 years old at the time and knew nothing of the relationship between that teacher and his mother. All he knew was that that teacher was loved by everyone -she treated everyone really well, was good at her job and very nurturing to her young pupils. The only person she treated harshly was him. The only conclusion he could draw from that limited information was that he must be a bad person in some way. He must have deserved to be treated that way, because she wouldn't have treated him badly if he hadn't deserved it.

If we're treated badly by someone, and they treat everyone that way, they seem bad-tempered and angry and critical with everyone, people soon agree that it's that person's problem. If we're treated badly by someone who is, with everyone else, kind and gentle and encouraging, then we, and everyone else around, are likely to assume it's our fault.

That's why the misunderstandings that are at the very roots of a symptom, condition or issue often involve someone we remember as being a good or nice person. Many people assume that the roots are more likely to involve someone we remember as nasty, but that is very rarely the case.

Knock-on effects

There were seeds of doubt planted in his young mind that there was something badly wrong with him, and once we have those kinds of doubts about ourselves, we can use the most tenuous links to nurture and tend to those seeds. Every time someone doesn't say hello to us, it's because we're bad – even if they simply didn't see us. Every time something is broken, or stolen – every time someone is hurt or upset, then it's because we did something wrong.

We can't remember doing anything and we didn't intend to, but we were around at the time, so it was probably us. After all, we didn't intend to do anything wrong the first time, but there was clear evidence that time that we caused all the harm.

We learn to stop trusting ourselves to be able to achieve our objectives. We learn to expect that, however hard we try, however much we want to do the right thing, to be good, we're simply going to fail because, deep down, there's something rotten inside us that 'all the perfumes of Arabia will not sweeten...'

Some of this processing may be conscious, in that we may remember going through those kinds of thoughts and coming to those kinds of conclusions. More often, though, it seems that the processing starts out that way, out in the open, and then finds its way into the background.

Pat: *If this incident was one that he had thought about from time to time, as an adult, did he view it the same way before treatment as after?*

Me: Here again in Bill's own words: -

> *Mostly before the treatment I avoided thinking about the event as it was surrounded by feelings of rejection and humiliation. I had mostly thought that the event was my fault for trying to be 'special' by dropping my thing off early.*

> *However, after treatment I realised that the teacher's reaction was not proportionate. A quiet word with me or asking my mum to stop me was a reasonable response. However, I also found out some years later that my mum and the teacher had not got on but not connected to 2 things together. I have also spoken to my mum since and she explained that the teacher had 'bullied' her until my Mum realised that was what she was doing and not allowed it to continue. So the reason the teacher had shouted at me was because of her relationship with my mum and not me.*

In general, a client can, consciously as well as subconsciously, re-process such a memory in a new and different way, so that the same incident then has a totally different interpretation and a refreshingly healthier, happier set of knock-on effects.

The subconscious mind is a closed book that we can't analyse directly. We're on a train and can see where we set off from, and the towns and countryside that we travel through, except that, from time to time, it all goes dark. Then we emerge from the other side of a hill or from under a river or a narrow channel of the sea. That section of the journey gives us no direct information about where we've been, but by looking at the map, at what we last saw before the darkness, at what we first saw when the light returned, and checking our watch to see how long had elapsed without that view from the window, we can be pretty sure that we went in a fairly straight line at a fairly steady speed through a tunnel.

It's that kind of analysis of information we can gain from the conscious mind that gives us a few ideas of what might have been going on behind the scenes for information that the conscious mind can't remember. We create some theories and then, in the best of scientific methods, we gain as much evidence as we can, and specifically, search for anything that might disprove our theory.

If we fail to disprove it, then we gain more and more confidence that we're on the right track. If we are on the right track, then we start to see more and more landmarks that confirm our route. As we get nearer to our destination, then we begin to get some improvements in the unwelcome, undesirable and even unhealthy symptom.

Follow-on memories

As he grew a little older, it started to be a treat for Bill to go to a cafe with his mum, for some special, one-to-one time. Those trips would often end badly. This was the first memory of being ill in some way that seemed to be connected with food.

It may have served two purposes.

If his subconscious had created a belief, or even a strong suspicion, that he was a bad person, then it would make sense that he didn't deserve that special time with Mum, so being ill would spoil if for him, so he couldn't enjoy it.

If his subconscious believed he was bad, but needed to know that he wasn't 'that bad', then it would set up experiences to test it out. If he was ill and was looked after, then he clearly wasn't 'that bad'. He would have those reassuring experiences at fairly regular intervals, and always got the self-affirming nurturing response.

When he got older, his relationship with his mother began to be gradually replaced with more equal relationships with his peers. If there was, in fact, a deep, subconscious need for reassurance, then that need continued to be met by the sympathetic responses and the special treatment he got whenever he was ill.

It's quite easy to expect that many mothers will instinctively look after their child, physically and emotionally, whenever they are ill, however often they are ill, however mild or severe are the symptoms and however old they are. The average acquaintance or friend might not be quite so eager to continually change their plans, disrupt their own social life, put up with their own disappointment unless the person is very ill.

He suffered massively when he inadvertently ate something containing gluten. His life was restricted. He had to carry enough food with him every day as gluten-free food isn't generally available from the corner shop or local cafe.

There is no way that anyone would want, or be able to, at will, create the kind of symptoms he had. The process was all subconscious.

His symptoms started to get worse.

Gluten entered the picture

A pattern started to emerge and, with help from his partner, he began to exclude certain types of foods from his diet. By the time we started treatment, it had stabilised and had been stable for a few years. As long as he stayed away totally from even the tiniest amounts of gluten, he was physically healthy and symptom-free.

Treatment progressing

Further sessions included more information to be re-examined. I got confirmation that some reinterpretation had taken place, that further processing had happened as a result, and that all was proceeding well.

We left a few weeks for more of that processing to happen and I got several texts during that time that spoke of gluten-laden food eaten the day before and no ill effects experienced.

The texts I received:

I've eaten half a small slice of bread and it's not made me poorly. I'm so excited! Thanks again. You're my hero!

Thought you might like 2 know that yesterday I had a chip butty and a beer and I'm still ok! You're my hero!

Something had clearly changed.

After the sessions where we tied up some loose ends, I checked for any missed stray roots. None could be found and he was able to steadily increase his intake of toast, scones, biscuits, and even beer that had previously been such a poison to him.

The investigation had passed a crucial point. It seemed like we had found the key and unlocked the door. He was happy to give it a few weeks to see if he felt ok to eat more, and if he remained well after eating it.

We did a further session and everything that I could think of to check on seemed to be checking out totally.

I was happy, at that stage, to sign off his treatment, and that was in spring 2008.

To date, we've had no further treatment sessions for this gluten intolerance and he remains able to eat standard food containing gluten without any of his previous symptoms.

He has been happy to tell friends and acquaintances about his new state of health and his now widened diet. Others have been surprised to see him eating something from a packet, something shop-bought and main-stream - not gluten-free. And 6 years on, he is still able to eat freely without any of those adverse effects.

Since treatment, he and his wife have been able to go to France for a holiday. Previously, that would have been much more expensive and a huge effort as gluten-free food would have to be bought and home-baking would have been needed prior to the trip. It just wouldn't have been viable. Instead, he was able to enjoy some authentic crusty French bread.

I offered to mix up the causal incident about that teacher with a few others that people were able to tell me details about, so it couldn't be linked with any particular client – and include some that don't relate to the people whose stories I've told – and have at least one person's story that doesn't have any real-life details about the cause - so there wouldn't be any way anyone would be able to work out which cause was linked to which person.

But Bill and his wife pointed out that that would dilute the message, which is a powerful one that needs telling. As long as his name is disguised and no other identifying details are included, then only people they have already told the story to will have any idea who is the subject of this real-life story.

This isn't a scientific paper demonstrating proof that would stand up against peer review. Instead, it's meant to give some ideas for people to consider alongside some anecdotal evidence. One of my aims is to give people a reason to do some scientific research if the story that comes across has enough to excite the imagination of scientists in appropriate fields. My other aim is to demonstrate my own experiences of the potential benefits of LCH on physical ailments.

CHAPTER 14

It is only your own mind that can change anything and you cannot trick it into happening

The nudge that I needed

Bill and I have bumped into each other a number of times since 2008, and from time to time, he mentioned the subject of his treatment and asked after progress of my second book. I had to report that Book 2 wasn't actually progressing, and hadn't been given any of my time for many months. He seemed sad to hear that.

I've felt, over the years, that the story of LCH needs to be told to anyone who will listen. I've long believed that it has the potential to help where traditional western medicine has drawn a blank. I've hoped that this kind of therapy would result in more and more people recovering that quality of life from illnesses and conditions that medicines and surgery have not yet managed to cure.

What I hadn't picked up until quite recently is that people I have treated over the years have also felt the same. I had already interviewed several people and drafted initial versions of their LCH story. Some have checked in with me to see how things are progressing and I hadn't, until recently, considered that they might actually care about other people benefitting too.

That has been the single most powerful prod that has shifted my second book from the bottom of a seemingly endless to-do list up to very near the top. Now, it gets my time, my attention and my energy whenever the higher priorities of eating, sleeping, treating clients and a little bit of 'me-time' are satisfied for the day.

So a huge thank you to the people with the gluten intolerance, the nail-biting habit, the smoking habit and the eating/weight/food issue - ex-LCH-clients of mine, ex-sufferers who have offered or agreed to their story being told and to those who have enquired into the progress of Book2.

The end of treatment – the wider effects begin

When I treated Bill in 2008, I had no idea there was anything else bothering him except the gluten allergy. As far as I knew, he was otherwise healthy and happy. From what he said and what I observed, that's how it seemed to me. I got no clue about any other issue until he mentioned something to me about adjusting to life without the allergy, and that was probably a couple of years later.

For 4 or 5 years, he has been living a different kind of life, adjusting to no longer being ill if he wasn't extremely careful about what he ate, adjusting to eating what everyone else was eating. Instead of people feeling sorry for him, he found people celebrating with him. He was free of the severe food intolerance and could now eat all those foods that he had previously been craving.

But that's when he started to notice that he didn't feel quite as good as he had thought he would. He was happy to be able to eat freely and without fear, but something was unsettling him.

An idea began to form, progressing from a vague awareness in the back of his mind, evolving into a clear recognition. He realised that he hadn't just enjoyed people feeling sorry for him and cooking for him. He had really, really needed that. He didn't know why, he just knew he had needed it.

From the spring of 2008, he had had to begin to learn how to live without that special treatment.

He started to find that various memories were coming back to him, and with each one, he was able to see it in a different light. With the new understanding gained from his treatment, each of those memories seemed to take on a new meaning. Those new meanings allowed him to grow stronger, gain more belief in himself, feel better about himself, and maybe need a bit less sympathy.

When I met him in the spring of 2012, a clearer picture was beginning to emerge and things were slowly and steadily improving. There seemed to be a number of areas that were causing him problems in his daily life, and he was beginning to find that some of those problems were starting to reduce, but there was a sense of unfinished business. He continued to make progress for another year or so.

He contacted me in April 2013 and came to see me. He seemed to be struggling with something, wanting to talk but finding it very difficult. He had been mentally beating himself up for about 25 years, and he was still beating himself up when he walked in to my office that day.

He had been so nervous about facing up to his demons. He knew consciously that there might be a resolution to it, but he had no idea what that resolution might involve, and even worse, there might not be one at all. His subconscious was giving him a clear message, though.

The message he had been getting from his subconscious was loud as well as clear.

"This is it! I can't do any more. If you don't resolve this one, then you'll have to learn to live with it for the rest of your life. You know which incident you need to look at. It's up to you now."

He knew which incident it was. It was the one that had come into his mind when I treated him in 2008, but he hadn't been able to face it then.

In his words: -

During that first treatment, I saw the memory and thought 'I really hope this doesn't lead there. It's no good thinking about it now and they can't be connected, so ignore it and don't go there'.

He had told himself, his conscious mind, to get back to playing his part in treatment, leaving his subconscious to work with me without his influence, but his subconscious might have interpreted his conscious reaction to that memory as an instruction that that incident was off the agenda.

I didn't know anything about that incident or that inner 'conversation' at that time.

In 2013, he had to make that choice again, and this time he knew he had to face it.

He took a deep breath.

He took several.

He started to speak.

He described a memory from when he had been 6 years old, a painful memory filled, for him, with guilt and remorse. It emerged, as we discussed it further, that the memory had been with him from time to time throughout his childhood. As the months and years passed, experiences and lessons were learnt in the normal way. One side effect of some of those normal learning experiences was to add a whole new level of understanding to the memory of the incident that had happened when he had been 6 years old. A sense of unease had started to grow.

It grew, and grew.

Eventually, by the time he had reached the age of 12, the unease had turned into an unbearable urge to confess. He chose people he knew and trusted and went to them for advice. They confirmed that what he had done at 6 years old was something he shouldn't do, he really shouldn't do.

With the skills I've been using since 2006, I was able to spot a detail that he, and the people he had gone to for advice, had missed. What he had done was something that a 12 year old shouldn't do, mustn't do – but there are no circumstances, no circumstances at all, that would make it a wrong thing to do at 6 years old.

We took quite a long time reviewing his story from all angles and I spotted the detail that made it all make sense. A sensitive, caring, conscientious person couldn't possibly have done something so awful that he was convinced it meant that he was an abomination.

It couldn't be as he remembered it.

It couldn't be as he had interpreted it.

It wasn't.

It was as if a simple black and white pencil drawing had been made at the time when he was 6 years old. Then, as the months and years unfolded, layer upon layer of extra colour, detail and meaning had been added. The picture that eventually emerged was an oil painting full of horror.

Then, all the earlier sketches were lost and the only one that could be examined and studied, analysed and evaluated, was the full colour version. Then, the jury of the just and true agreed on their verdict – guilty as charged.

But on that day of revelation, in my office in April 2013, I found the original sketch. I used my LCH skills to remove layer upon layer of old paint and together, we reviewed the pencil drawing in all its innocence and simplicity. It seemed that well-meaning, understandable but totally fictional theories and erroneous assumptions had created all the subsequent terror that had haunted him for more than 2 decades.

Once he was able to see the incident in context, he found a sense of relief grow within him. It was a simple story of childhood innocence, with no need for any guilt or any remorse.

As he drove home that day, he felt a weight begin to lift from his shoulders. By the time he got home it had gone!

He described it as being like when a building is being demolished. There is a lot of preparation work, with explosives being placed in strategic places, connected to a central control button - and then the area is cleared. When everyone is out of the vicinity, the button is pushed.

Then there's a moment when nothing happens.

Then there's a bit of noise and smoke.

And then it starts.

The building begins to collapse into itself, slowly at first, maybe cascading through all the levels or floors. Then it gains momentum so that, suddenly, on the site where there had been a building, slightly damaged, there is suddenly, in its place, a pile of rubble and a pall of smoke and, if the job has gone to plan, nothing remaining from the old structure.

And that all happens, from start to finish, in moments, with the final stages as swift and complete as a dislodged house of cards.

That's what he experienced. Just like the way we can find ourselves watching such a demolition with fascination, he had found himself watching all his own unhappy history and tangle of misunderstandings unravel before his eyes. Something that had been an ugly part of his life, not wanted, a blot on his own landscape, was removed. It left a bit of clearing up to do, some dust and rubble to remove, but that was much easier once that demolition work had been completed.

In a similar way to Clare's' five-decade-long plate-clearing habit quite dramatically disappearing one day, Bill found that those feelings left him in minutes and the behaviour changes from 25 years of habits were completed in a matter of a few days. It needed a bit of time, but not that much.

The day after the visit to my office in April 2013, he was at work, having a catch-up with colleagues and finding the conversation going along very familiar lines. He was talking about his latest D.I.Y. project, how much work was involved, how complicated and difficult it all was, how tired he was feeling....

This time, though, he noticed something. It was as if he was observing from the sidelines at the same time as he was getting involved in the conversation. He saw how he was inviting the others to feel sorry for him by painting that kind of picture and he didn't want that pity. This time, he found himself including comments about how much he was enjoying a lot of the tasks and describing the immense satisfaction he was gaining from the results of his home-improvement projects.

So right from the very next day, he had started to notice a change. The need for sympathy was gone and he was finding his behaviour changing to fit with a different kind of need, to socialise, to share, to enjoy the banter with his peers, his colleagues.

As with Cathy who now feels like she's never been a smoker, he feels like how he is now is totally normal. It would feel alien to invite sympathy, and when he occasionally notices opportunities to 'milk' the situation, the thought he has now is 'well, why would I want to do that?' He has the memory of what it was like but no need for it any more.

It feels like a dramatic change because he knows on one level how much his life was different before, but at the same time, now it feels normal, it feels right. A totally different way of behaving around other people – not courting sympathy – suddenly felt normal just days after the opposite had been his constant state for 25 years!!!

By the time we got chance to catch up again in November and December, for a meeting and a couple of phone calls, he had pieced together a huge portion of the jigsaw. His conscious scientific mind had needed to go through that exercise and make sure it all fitted together. Any gaps or anomalies would need to be resolved before he could be sure that all the dots joined up.

He could see that the guilt and remorse had been so painful that he had needed regular reassurance. As long as people felt sorry for him and cooked for him, he knew he couldn't be that bad. His self-esteem was so low because of what he believed he had done. When people gave him treats, made him special food, it didn't make him feel like he was on a pedestal – it just lifted him up from the gutter so he could feel he was just about on a level with everyone else.

As long as he had the pain and discomfort and disruption to his life, deprived of many types of foods, fearful of having eaten any gluten, then Bill was serving his sentence for the 'crime' he had believed he'd committed.

The gluten allergy, the restricted diet, the fear of even traces of gluten causing severe and painful digestive disasters, the sympathy of others, the efforts that others made to make sure he got food that was safe to eat, all of this was medicating his real pain, the raw pain of the evil that he believed he had done.

Since the session in April 2013, he has become so free of all of that pain that he has been able to look back on it all from a different perspective. He could still clearly remember what the experience had been like during all those years when food had been making him ill. He also knew a period of time of raw pain without the allergy-side-effects moderating it for him.

Before he came to see me, he hadn't connected the guilt or the need for people to feel sorry for him in any way with the gluten. All he knew was that he felt great if someone cooked for him and particularly if anyone felt sorry for him.

Before the full resolution emerged, he believes his subconscious had been doing the best for him. If he had had to choose between the raw pain and the medicated pain, moderated by the allergy, he would have definitely chosen to keep the allergy. The mental/ emotional guilt and remorse were being kept under control, medicated, soothed, softened, mitigated by the secondary effects of his allergy.

To illustrate to me just what he was comparing in making that choice, he asked me to imagine or maybe remember having a tummy bug that was, at its worst, so severe that you wouldn't even consider going out of the house. As you got better, you were still a bit wobbly so you made sure you didn't go far from where you knew there was a toilet.

Imagine living with that for many years with no end in sight.

You couldn't let it rule your life.

You couldn't stay at home forever, just in case.

You never knew when it was going to strike but you had to live with it and get on with it as best you could.

With Bill, it got easier once the foods to be avoided had been identified and he'd stabilised his diet, but someone could always change a recipe or something could, at any time, get inadvertently contaminated, so it could still happen.

Before he got to that more stable state, it could and did happen. At any time, in any place, he would find himself with only enough warning to get to the toilet if there was one available nearby. Once stabilised, it was much rarer but it could still happen.

**Imagine living like that for years with no hope
of a cure.**

Then imagine how bad the guilt, the remorse, the
raw pain must have been if, looking back on it all,
he could see the allergy as definitely the lesser of
two evils.

Sometimes, when I'm explaining to prospective clients
that I believe the subconscious is always doing its best
for us, they look at their own symptom and ask me
how that could possibly be for their own good. Bill has
looked at the bigger picture and has no doubt that
even the worst of times that came along with the gluten
allergy were the better option. The worst of that ever-
present and unpredictable 'tummy bug', the fear of,
and the experience of, that literal gut reaction, was a
lesser pain, a lesser evil, a lesser distress than the raw
pain of guilt and remorse and of not knowing just what
kind of person he really was.

It's clear to me just how great a demon it must have
been to have haunted him for 25 years and held him
firmly in its control all that time.

And he is now free of both evils.

He was treated for one symptom, the gluten, and at the
time, neither he nor I knew of any connection it might
have with any deeper issues. He remembers clearly
being given the memory of that incident at 6 years old
when we got to that stage of treatment but he had
wished and hoped he wouldn't have to face it then.

Some people's symptoms are resolved without any relevant memories coming back to them. Some people have a memory that they connect with the symptom. Some, like Bill, have a significant memory that is their 'skeleton in the cupboard' and they don't want to think about it, let alone talk about it.

When clients refer to any of those kinds of incidents that might be part of the development of the symptom, in some cases, might even be the causal incident, I explain that, even in that case, there must be some aspect of it, some specific detail, something that was not exactly how it had been remembered.

It seems to me that Bill's conscious mind and his subconscious mind each held a different key to fully resolving the gluten allergy and every one of the reasons why he had needed it.

The door would only unlock and open up to the sunshine once both keys had been turned. His conscious and subconscious mind both needed to play their own role. Neither part of his mind, on its own, could fully resolve it because each part of his mind had contributed in its own way to creating his mental prison sentence. Only when both keys were in place and turned could he walk out as a free man.

Bill also believes that you can't fake a solution. People can say 'you don't need to worry about that' or 'why are you worrying about that?' without that providing anything more than a temporary alleviation. He just had to get it fully resolved. He had needed to see that specific detail. He couldn't possibly have known at 6 years old, couldn't possibly have thought like an adult at that age. Reassurance can make things a little better temporarily, but a full resolution needs that one key fact to slot into place.

He also now believes his relationship with his subconscious is much stronger, and that strength was already starting to build by the time we had completed his treatment in 2008. When he had first started getting a feeling that it was ok to eat a little bit of gluten, that it wouldn't make him ill, he knew he would be ok. His wife wasn't so sure.

Once his treatment was completed, he wanted to celebrate by having his first full non-gluten-free meal in a restaurant, to mark the occasion in style. His wife wanted that first meal to be in the safety of their own home. She was so nervous, convinced he would, at any moment, rush from the table to the toilets. She couldn't believe that the 'tummy bug' was so completely gone. He knew. He was fine. He had had no doubts about it.

He has been learning more and more about that powerful relationship between the conscious and subconscious mind. They can work together as a team, in tune with each other, complementing each other, recognising each other's skills and how to bring the best out in each other. It's that kind of benefit that Bill has gained from his hypnotherapy treatment and all the follow-on conscious work he has been doing.

He has lost the allergy and resolved a huge chunk of the reason why he had needed the allergy. We don't know, as yet, whether there is another subconscious layer to explore or whether the resolution to all the remaining issues is now in the pipeline.

If there isn't another layer, then he has the ability, the motivation, the strength, the energy to climb hill after hill until he reaches his summit.

If there is subconscious work to do, then that's my speciality. I will update the story in a further book or a later edition of this one, if appropriate, and if Bill wants to continue to share his experiences and understanding as things continue to develop.

Some of Bill's thoughts

I have been trying really hard to describe the strange feeling of being completely different and it feeling normal/OK. I know how much you like your analogies so this is the best I have come up with is something like moving house. You know that you now live in a new place and have known that you will for some time so you are used to the idea but there is one night where you sleep in the old house and then the next night you sleep in the new one and will never go back to the old house again.

You fit all your things into the house and start to make it your home. Within a few days all the things that you need are unpacked and put out. The house feels a little unusual as you get used to it but very quickly it starts to feel like home as you have brought all your things with you. Considering how much is different it is a huge change but we adapt to it quite quickly and it starts to feel normal.

Another good example is going to stay in a caravan or narrow boat. You take the core of everything with you but you are in a completely new place and you don't know where to find anything like shops etc which takes some getting used to but with experience and help you can learn those things quickly and settle down to enjoy your holiday. It always feels like coming "home" from a day out, even after that first night.

*This is kind of how it felt to have that sudden change. Everything looked very different, like taking sunglasses off but **the core of who I am stays and so it still feels normal**, you can remember where you used to live but you know that you don't live there anymore. Sometimes on autopilot you may go back down your old street before realising that you don't live there anymore but you soon become used to your new location.*

It's not like it never happened as I remember the feeling and motivation to get people to feel sorry for me but the drive is no longer there. Some habits have taken a bit longer to change, like learning how to get to the shops in a new house or blowing a fuse and not knowing where the fuse box is!

However, virtually from the moment I walked out of your door that day it was gone. I have had a few times where the memories have come back, but instead of haunting me I have been able to think about them and re evaluate them, which I could never do before. It is almost like my subconscious is just checking in and asking "do we still agree with the conclusions from this?"

Like if you ever have got lost reading a map, you think that you are in one place and then you notice a feature or landmark that doesn't fit in with where you think that you are. You stop, reassess your location and then carry on having taken the new information on board. Every time I have done something like that there is a revelation moment where you think "Oh, of course, that makes a lot more sense, how could I have thought I was in that different location?" but you just use the new information to direct you more accurately and get on with travelling to your destination.

When you came to see me I think that I was in a kind of crisis as my gluten allergy was not giving me what I needed but I didn't know how to change to get what I needed. It also stemmed from a memory that I had consciously over 25 year locked away as I was ashamed of it and it was very painful to think about. Every time I had thought about it I had added the new experiences onto it so I then remembered it as if I had done it as a much older person who didn't have the innocence of a child.

Even though in the first treatment I didn't fully unlock everything, because I wasn't consciously willing to face that root memory, I was able to change a lot, such as my gluten allergy. It wasn't until my wife pointed out to me that I was still trying to get sympathy and that she thought that was the root cause of my gluten allergy too that I made the link and was able to come for more treatment (although it was basically counselling rather than LCH but it was communication with my subconscious) to remove the blockage and be truly free of it.

I have also been thinking how amazing we are as humans to have developed a way for our brains to control our bodies but also to not have to think about doing it all the time. We know scientifically that the brain controls a lot of our bodies as the chemicals and nerves that create changes are all controlled from the brain. However, would we be able to achieve most of what we do as humans if we had to think all the time about breathing or maintaining our body temperature or digesting food?

It is extremely clever that we have developed a part of the brain that controls all of that without us having to think about it. However, it is all one brain and there are cross overs. The subconscious part of our brains can also talk to the conscious parts and send signals such as "I can't maintain body temperature, put a jumper on or go inside.....".

The subconscious part of our brains is also a simple processor, processing huge amounts of data all the time and is not capable of more abstract thinking and relies on our conscious part of our brains to do that. It is almost like having a guardian angel sitting on your shoulder all the time looking out for you, even simple things like "you have forgotten something" (we all know that nagging feeling, even if we can't think what we have forgotten).

However, you can never trick your own mind. You have to truly find what the root cause is and deal with it. Some people will do this entirely subconsciously but others like myself will want to know what is going on and understand the process. Also in my case I needed to consciously re evaluate the original incident and honestly truly believe that I had not committed an unforgivable crime.

Until I had done that, until Mary had pointed out I could not have possibly thought like an adult at 6 years old, until I saw my own children innocently doing the same things that I did, I never could truly believe what I had done was OK. If I had never plucked up the courage to open up and look at the incident I would never have been free.

I knew that I had a choice. Keep living like the way I had or risk looking at it and re assessing it with someone else to see if there was a way through. I did not know if there would be a way through. I thought that I may have to learn to live with it but I also felt that there was something wrong with my interpretation of it. I was not easy but I decided that I wanted to change and so faced it. I am very, very pleased that I did.

I think that this is an important message for those considering LCH. **LCH cannot trick you into thinking anything. It can only highlight where a problem started and allow you, perhaps with some guidance from the practitioner to re evaluate the experience and the outcomes that you drew from it. Nothing will change unless you believe the new evaluation. It is only your own mind that can change anything and you cannot trick it into happening.**

A lot of people ask me if it was like tricking you into believing something or if you were not aware of what was happening. This is definitely not true. It is led by your subconscious but it is still your mind and as required your subconscious will make you aware of parts of the conversation or will prompt memories that you may have to deal with. It is never, ever out of your control and you will never be brain washed. LCH cannot trick you into believing something that you don't think is true.

Not just Bill

Treatment can often lead to improvements in other areas. Because people tend to learn, as treatment progresses, that LCH digs up the roots of the weeds rather than simply chop off the unsightly greenery above the soil, when they return to some of the later sessions, some report other improvements and attribute them to LCH.

They've made no other changes during that time frame, so have nothing else to thank for the benefits. They feel, instinctively, that something deep within them has been fixed. They get a kind of feeling, a strange sense that something good has taken place, that a dilemma they hadn't known that they had has been resolved in the background.

When we turn off the extractor fan over the hob in the kitchen, if it's been on for some time, we can get a sense of relief that we didn't previously know we needed. People have described feeling better about themselves, a peace of mind, a sense that that previous inevitable certainty that 'it must be my fault' has gone, and gone for good.

Me: Pat and Chris – what are the main messages?

Pat: *That even if we don't want to find the answer in the mind, for whatever reason, it's worth looking, just in case. I can't imagine anyone outside of the world of LCH expecting that Bill would be able to eat gluten without getting ill when all that took place was a kind of talking therapy.*

      After all, it was a physical symptom. It wasn't something we have any conscious control over. This form of talking therapy resolved the underlying cause, which turned out to have been a subconscious underlying cause. So did the subconscious create the symptom in the first place, and then, when it wasn't needed any more, did the subconscious undo the symptom?

Me: That's the best way I can make sense of it all in my own mind. Maybe other people have some other explanation for what Bill experienced. I'd be very interested to hear what other theories could explain it all.

Chris: *And what about all the other physical symptoms and illnesses where the only available medical intervention is symptom relief, with no cure available as yet? Might LCH be another avenue to consider? It could be used, not as an alternative, but as a complementary therapy alongside the medical treatments. It seems like it has the potential to unlock the door and free some people from their suffering.*

And again, like Cathy who lost her long-standing sense of guilt, the shining light for me is the wider or deeper change. Bill had needed people to feel sorry for him, even though he wasn't aware that he did. That need must have got in his way so much. Life must be so much simpler for him now.

I wonder if my smoking and my weight are doing something similar for me. I might also have much to gain, in addition to an improved state of physical health, if I get help to resolve those eating and smoking cravings at the root rather than continuing to spend my time, money and energy on lopping off the branches using my own willpower and other measures focussed directly on the cravings and addictions.

I think the main message I'm going to take away is to challenge my own pessimistic expectations, even if most other people would agree with those predictions.

LCH and the subconscious mind have significantly improved the lives of Clare and Cathy, Steve and Bill.

They clearly won't be the only ones who have benefitted.

CHAPTER 15

I smile and agree with my subconscious that she and I are OK just as we are

And now, humour me please, as I take just a little time for some unsolicited self-revelation...

My clients have been happy to share, anonymously, some of their individual experiences. With their stories and my explanations and my interpretations of LCH and the subconscious in relation to those stories almost complete, I find myself drawn to say a bit more about my own experience as a client.

Here is a little glimpse of what I can thank LCH for....

My Mum was scared of her own shadow and lived in everyone else's. My Dad lived in a very small private world, grunting a broad-Yorkshire Yes or No or at most, a two or three word answer to anyone who wanted to pass the time of day with him or get to know him. People tried, but not many, outside of our immediate family, could get through to either of them.

My own root cause or causes, possibly the model boat I'd 'fixed' (see 'What if it really is... ?'), possibly others I still don't remember but nevertheless have been resolved by my subconscious, have recently unlocked some long-barred rooms in my mental sanctuary. The way I had learnt to live would have fitted better in the traditional Japanese culture of deference, lowered gaze, quiet unless invited or required by a superior or elder to answer a question.

Mum and Dad were a big influence on me in those early formative years with no nursery or playgroup or childminder socialising to dilute their ways of relating to the world. But that doesn't determine who I am because my brothers had the same upbringing as I did and, as far as I know, felt far more comfortable around others than I have been.

More recently, I find I look people in the eye as an equal, with a smile that comes from knowing 'You're definitely OK and always have been, and, do you know what, I'm actually OK too now.'

A bit like Pat and Chris with that food and eating debate, those who have always known they're OK will wonder why the big deal. Those who, like me, have felt socially awkward will recognise the relief of time on our own after a long and draining event that others enjoy. For those of us who feel, or 'know' we're not OK, we feel like we only just cope if we put all our attention and energy into saying and doing the right thing.

One to one is easier. One in a crowd at a dance event is a breeze. One in a group all interacting with each other is a constant and exhausting juggling or plate-spinning act. I'm not sure if there is still more work I need to do, more treatment I need to receive, but things seem to be improving still from time to time. Maybe I need more treatment or maybe all I want and need to progress is already in the pipeline. Maybe one day, I'll fully believe that I am just right as I am, and that my own unique self and the contribution I make to the world is just as valid as anyone else's. Maybe, eventually, I'll become fully, totally and comfortably true to myself.

I know some lovely people and enjoy time with them, but for years have struggled and strived to reach a level of being OK company for them.

Now, from time to time, more and more often recently, I actually smile, feel a sense of relief, notice where that tension comes from and agree with my subconscious that she and I are OK just as we are. We smile even more as we let that tension go so those lovely folk can actually get through.

As I write this, I can feel a sense of contradiction or contrariness (not a coincidence my name is Mary). In some aspects, I have confidence, a self-belief, and ability to speak up for myself, to disagree with received wisdom and many more simple examples that show opposite traits within me.

There is a paradox here. We can be gifted and challenged at the same time, in apparently similar areas. The mind and the brain are both so complex and what seems similar to the conscious mind might actually require totally different subconscious processing and the firing of totally different parts of the brain.

I have a warm and comforting feeling that I'm definitely OK, that I always have been and always will be. I've worried needlessly for so long, about what I've said and done, about what I might say and do in the future.

Like probably just about everyone else in the world, I put my foot in it from time to time...

And that created my old song...

The Animals' heartfelt

'Please don't let me be misunderstood'

But that is now being replaced by some different ones like the message I'm starting to send between my conscious and subconscious mind – and which I'm also now beginning to send to those lovely people I care about...

Randy Newman's innocent, playful, smiling 'You've got a friend in me'.

CHAPTER 16

Maybe we could find a reason not to unquestioningly trust the predictions of those who confidently tell us there is no cure

An afterthought or two...

Chris: *Do we need to carry on preferring to find out that the cause of any ailment is purely physical? Would we gain from questioning that idea? Can we add to our resources with complementary therapies rather than limit ourselves to purely what the doctor advises?*

   And if so, how can we encourage people to get comfortable with psychological or subconscious causes so that they widen their search for solutions?

   How do you feel about needing treatment for so many aspects, psychological and physical within yourself?

Me: For myself, I feel fine about it because I see the subconscious mind as just as remote from my control and willpower as my gallbladder, my thyroid gland and my kidneys, so I don't need to feel like I should be able to pull myself together and just get over it.

I don't feel undermined by it. It doesn't feel like I'm weak willed or weak minded because I couldn't fix it for myself. It just feels like something isn't working properly and I need the help of someone trained in the appropriate field.

There are only 4 cases described here so it's not statistically significant. It's purely anecdotal, but surely it includes some unexpected results from a talking therapy only a few have heard of and even fewer have trained in and practise. So is it worth studying further?

I saw a TV programme about dementia and other forms of mental deterioration in old age. It was screened a year or two ago so my memory of it is a bit vague on the details. Scientists were devoting their whole life's work to specific research into smaller and smaller areas, the DNA, genes etc but it looked to me like there was a much greater benefit that had been caused by a behavioural approach, by simply treating people differently.

A group of elderly people were invited to take part in an experiment and spent a few weeks in a residential setting where, in spite of their advanced ages and some physical and medical conditions getting in their way, they were expected to carry their own suitcases in from the coach, make their own beds, cook for themselves and generally stretch beyond what was normally asked from them in their normal care home environments. They were invited to engage in wider and deeper ways, physically, mentally and emotionally, with their environment and with each other.

In just a few weeks, their behaviour had changed, their mobility had improved, aches and pains had reduced, concentration had increased and mood had lifted.

Maybe my memory of the program was distorted. Maybe my interpretation of the relative findings was biased, but it seemed to me that the last word, the summary, the way forward was given by one of those scientists optimistically going back to the lab and the ever stronger microscope, saying "maybe not in my lifetime but I'm going to carry on because I believe the answer is here if I just keep digging deeper". There seemed to be no suggestion that the behavioural research that showed such significant results would be pursued and developed and consolidated eventually into some new guidelines for how we treat people as they grow older.

This has been an account of anecdotal evidence of benefits gained together with some musings about how and why these people enjoyed the positive changes they experienced. These are my musings, my 'take' on a particular kind of therapy, my way of looking at the subconscious mind. These musings may be totally off the wall and my theories completely incorrect, but surely, some of the information here has surprised you. Surely some of the outcomes were ones that you, like Chris and Pat and Cathy and Bill, possibly also Clare and Steve, wouldn't have predicted.

The 4 generous case-study subjects and many more
reviewers, friends, colleagues, friends of friends,
and I all have a combined wish that working with
the subconscious mind, maybe in the form of LCH or
some other similar therapy, is considered before, or
at least, alongside, other forms of treatment that have
significant severe and long-lasting side effects.

**If medicine says 'it's incurable' or someone believes
'that's just how I am and I have to live with it', then
I hope that these few remarkable people and their
powerful stories lead to some different ideas being
at least considered.**

Again, I have a memory that illustrates it for me.
I remember a holiday on a barge, many years ago. It was
my job to open the locks and the swing bridges. One
day, I encountered a huge metal bridge and a man who
looked physically fit and strong. He was pushing and
tugging at the bridge and making no impression on it.

I added my almost insignificant extra strength to his in
case that might be enough to get it moving. It wasn't,
and I just leaned on the gate, in the sunshine, and
chatted with my new companion while we patiently
waited for the crews of our respective boats to moor
up and add their shoulders to the effort.

They hadn't yet arrived when I noticed that there was
some movement. It was extremely slight at first, almost
imperceptible, but it soon began to gain momentum.
Circumstances had conspired to provide an answer.
If we hadn't had to wait, then we would never have

learnt that a fairly small and physically slight and weak person as I was then, could move a heavy object that a much stronger person hadn't managed to push or pull along. All I did was lean against it. The bridge started to move when it was ready, at its own pace. It eventually gained its own momentum and continued its journey across the water with only a little bit of extra encouragement.

Maybe it's another allegorical hint not to underestimate the power of the subconscious.

Maybe we could also see it as a reason not to immediately and unquestioningly trust the predictions of those with the most apparently relevant knowledge and expertise and skills if they confidently tell us there is no cure.

I'm offering here some glimpses of life-changing treatments which, in comparison to the high-tech world of MRI scanning, surgery, gene therapy and the like, is small and understated, often and easily overlooked, like in the dementia documentary.

I believe it deserves more of our attention.

Think back to before you started to read about LCH. What did you expect?

If we don't expect to find a parking space, then we'll quickly give up trying to find one if there isn't one immediately visible. If we believe there's bound to be a space, that we always find one, in a car park of this size, there's definitely one somewhere, then we'll keep on looking until we spot the one hidden away in the corner or someone returns with their shopping and drives off leaving that space for us to drive in to.

So that's a happy result from expecting success and sadness or frustration from expecting the worst.

Let's celebrate placebo. To me, that's just another word for 'We don't know how or why it works yet. We just know that it does!' With spontaneous remission and treatment behaving as a catalyst for beneficial change, and even pure coincidence, let's enjoy and celebrate them all.

Whatever works, before we find out why and how it works, if the risks are small, predictable and manageable, let's reap the benefits.

When you first picked up this book, I wonder - what did you expect?

And now I wonder...

What do you expect... ?

Note from the Author

And now that my second book is complete, there still seems so much more to study and so much more to say. As long as I continue treating clients and learning more about LCH and the subconscious, I'll be continuing to write about how it all looks to me. From the moment the final version of book 2 is signed off, book 3 will be beginning to germinate.

If you want to have any input into that process, then I'd love to hear from you.

If you have questions about any of what you have just read and haven't yet read 'What if...', then please look there first. When you've read both books, please know that I appreciate any constructive feedback and any questions raised for you by what I've written and I'll do my best to respond as constructively as I can.

If you want more information about treatment or training, or if you wish to send me any feedback of your own, you will find my contact details via my website www.curativehypnotherapyyork.co.uk and the training college website is www.lesserian.co.uk

Cheers! – Salud! – Santé! – Salute! - Je via sano!

Mary Ratcliffe

www.ingramcontent.com/pod-product-compliance
Lightning Source LLC
Chambersburg PA
CBHW031150270326
41931CB00006B/215